Manual of
Clinical Periodontics

Manual of
Clinical Periodontics

Second Edition

Shantipriya Reddy
BDS MDS (Periodontia)
Professor and Head
Department of Periodontics
Dr Syamala Reddy Dental College, Hospital and Research Centre
Bengaluru, Karnataka, India

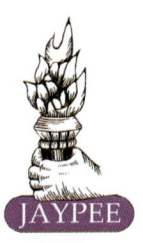

JAYPEE BROTHERS MEDICAL PUBLISHERS (P) LTD

New Delhi • London • Philadelphia • Panama

Jaypee Brothers Medical Publishers (P) Ltd

Headquarters

Jaypee Brothers Medical Publishers (P) Ltd
4838/24, Ansari Road, Daryaganj
New Delhi 110 002, India
Phone: +91-11-43574357
Fax: +91-11-43574314
Email: jaypee@jaypeebrothers.com

Overseas Offices

J.P. Medical Ltd
83 Victoria Street, London
SW1H 0HW (UK)
Phone: +44-2031708910
Fax: +02-03-0086180
Email: info@jpmedpub.com

Jaypee-Highlights Medical Publishers Inc
City of Knowledge, Bld. 237, Clayton
Panama City, Panama
Phone: +1 507-301-0496
Fax: +1 507-301-0499
Email: cservice@jphmedical.com

Jaypee Medical Inc
The Bourse
111 South Independence Mall East
Suite 835, Philadelphia, PA 19106, USA
Phone: +1 267-519-9789
Email: jpmed.us@gmail.com

Jaypee Brothers Medical Publishers (P) Ltd
17/1-B Babar Road, Block-B, Shaymali
Mohammadpur, Dhaka-1207
Bangladesh
Mobile: +08801912003485
Email: jaypeedhaka@gmail.com

Jaypee Brothers Medical Publishers (P) Ltd
Bhotahity, Kathmandu
Nepal
Phone: +977-9741283608
Email: kathmandu@jaypeebrothers.com

Website: www.jaypeebrothers.com
Website: www.jaypeedigital.com

© 2014, Jaypee Brothers Medical Publishers

The views and opinions expressed in this book are solely those of the original contributor(s)/author(s) and do not necessarily represent those of editor(s) of the book.

All rights reserved. No part of this publication may be reproduced, stored or transmitted in any form or by any means, electronic, mechanical, photocopying, recording or otherwise, without the prior permission in writing of the publishers.

All brand names and product names used in this book are trade names, service marks, trademarks or registered trademarks of their respective owners. The publisher is not associated with any product or vendor mentioned in this book.

Medical knowledge and practice change constantly. This book is designed to provide accurate, authoritative information about the subject matter in question. However, readers are advised to check the most current information available on procedures included and check information from the manufacturer of each product to be administered, to verify the recommended dose, formula, method and duration of administration, adverse effects and contraindications. It is the responsibility of the practitioner to take all appropriate safety precautions. Neither the publisher nor the author(s)/editor(s) assume any liability for any injury and/or damage to persons or property arising from or related to use of material in this book.

This book is sold on the understanding that the publisher is not engaged in providing professional medical services. If such advice or services are required, the services of a competent medical professional should be sought.

Every effort has been made where necessary to contact holders of copyright to obtain permission to reproduce copyright material. If any have been inadvertently overlooked, the publisher will be pleased to make the necessary arrangements at the first opportunity.

Inquiries for bulk sales may be solicited at: jaypee@jaypeebrothers.com

Manual of Clinical Periodontics

First Edition: 2011
Second Edition: **2014**

ISBN 978-93-5152-248-5

Printed at: Ajanta Offset & Packagings Ltd., New Delhi

Preface to the Second Edition

It gives me great pleasure to present the second edition of *Manual of Clinical Periodontics,* which is provided as add on with the textbook.

Conscious attempts have been made not to disturb the clarity and simplicity of the main text, which had gained immense popularity amongst the students.

Shantipriya Reddy

Preface to the First Edition

It gives me great pleasure to present the *Manual of Clinical Periodontics,* which is provided as an Add on with the textbook.

This manual was written with a purpose of helping the students to overcome various difficulties they come across while recording clinical case history, arriving at a proper diagnosis and executing various treatment procedures. The clarity and simplicity of the language adopted in the manual will benefit the students in understanding and applying the principles of clinical periodontics.

Manual is divided under the sections of case history format, clinical examination, diagnosis and treatment plan, periodontal instruments and instrumentation. They have been elaborated and presented with self-explanatory flow charts, clinical photographs and colored diagrams.

The *Manual of Clinical Periodontics* summarizes a vast branch of clinical periodontology in a nutshell, guiding the undergraduate students to a deeper insight into the subject. I hope this manual fulfills the need with which it is written, which will help the students, develop a better clinical acumen.

Shantipriya Reddy

Contents

Section 1: Case History Recording

1. **Case History Format** — 1
   - *Gingival Status* 2
2. **Recording Clinical Case History** — 4
   - *Key Stages of Case History Recording* 4
   - *History Recording* 4
   - *Clinical Evaluation, Diagnosis and Treatment Planning* 4
   - *Investigations* 15
   - *Prognosis* 15
   - *Clinical Factors Used in Determining Prognosis* 16
   - *Periodontal Treatment Plan* 17
   - *Treatment of Gingivitis* 18
   - *Chronic Periodontitis* 19
   - *Tissue Response to Periodontal Therapy* 19

Section 2: Instrumentation

3. **Periodontal Instruments and Instrumentation** — 21
   - *Parts of Periodontal Instruments* 21
   - *Classification of Periodontal Instruments* 21
   - *Diagnostic Instruments* 21
   - *Scaling and Root Planing Instruments* 23
   - *Supragingival Scalers* 23
   - *Subgingival Scalers* 24
   - *Subgingival Scaling and Root Planing Instruments* 25
   - *Advances in Root Planing Instruments* 25
   - *Principles of Periodontal Instrumentation* 26
   - *Recommended Position* 29
   - *Basic Positioning of the Patient's Head* 29
   - *Visibility, Illumination and Retraction* 29
   - *Transillumination* 30
   - *Condition of Instruments (Sharpness)* 30
   - *Maintaining a Clean Field* 30
   - *Instrument Stabilization* 31
   - *Instrument Activation* 32
   - *Lateral Pressure* 33
   - *Types of Stroke by Direction* 33

Section 3: Viva Voce

4.	Anatomy and Development of the Structures of Periodontium	37
5.	Biology of Periodontal Tissues	39
6.	Periodontal Structures in Aging Humans	45
7.	Classification Systems of Periodontal Diseases	46
8.	Epidemiology of Gingival and Periodontal Diseases	48
9.	Periodontal Microbiology	51
10.	Calculus and Other Etiological Factors	53
11.	Host Response: Basic Concepts	56
12.	Trauma from Occlusion	58
13.	Role of Systemic Diseases in the Etiology of Periodontal Diseases	61
14.	Oral Malodor	64
15.	Pathogenesis of Periodontal Diseases	65
16.	Periodontal Medicine	67
17.	Smoking and Periodontal Disease	68
18.	Host Modulation in Periodontal Therapy	69
19.	Defense Mechanism of Gingiva	70
20.	Gingival Inflammation	72
21.	Clinical Features of Gingivitis	73
22.	Gingival Enlargements	77
23.	Acute Gingival Infections	82
24.	Periodontal Diseases in Children and Young Adolescents	86
25.	Desquamative Gingivitis	88
26.	Periodontal Pocket	90
27.	Bone Loss and Patterns of Bone Destruction	94
28.	Chronic Periodontitis	96
29.	Aggressive Periodontitis	98
30.	Necrotizing Ulcerative Periodontitis, Refractory Periodontitis and Periodontitis as a Manifestation of Systemic Disease	100
31.	AIDS and the Periodontium	102
32.	Diagnosis of Periodontal Diseases	103
33.	Prognosis	105
34.	Related Risk Factors Associated with Periodontal Diseases	107
35.	Various Aids Including Advanced Diagnostic Aids	109
36.	Treatment Plan	112
37.	Rationale for Periodontal Treatment	113
38.	Periodontal Instrumentation	114
39.	Principles of Periodontal Instrumentation Including Scaling and Root Planing	118
40.	Plaque Control	124
41.	Principles of Periodontal Surgery	129
42.	Gingival Curettage	131
43.	Gingivectomy	133

44.	Periodontal Flap	135
45.	Osseous Surgery	138
46.	Mucogingival Surgery	144
47.	Furcation Involvement and its Management	149
48.	Pulpoperiodontal Problems	154
49.	Splints in Periodontal Therapy	156
50.	Dental Implants: Periodontal Considerations	158
51.	Maintenance Phase (Supportive Periodontal Treatment)	160
52.	Occlusal Evaluation and Therapy in the Management of Periodontal Disease	162
53.	The Role of Orthodontics as an Adjunct to Periodontal Therapy	164
54.	Periodontal-restorative Inter-relationship	166
55.	Drugs Used in Periodontal Therapy	168

Index   *173*

CHAPTER 1

SECTION 1: Case History Recording

Case History Format

Name: _____
Age: _____ Occupation: _____
Sex: _____ Address: _____
_____
OP No: _____ Date: _____
Chief Complaint: _____
_____
_____
History of Present Illness: _____
_____
_____

Past dental history:
   a. Frequency of dental visits:
   b. Date of last prophylaxis:
   c. Frequency of oral prophylaxis:
   d. History of previous dental treatment:

Family dental history:
   a. History of caries/periodontal disease:
   b. Unusual loss of teeth in parents or siblings:

Medical history:

Cardiac:
- Chest pain on exertion
- Palpitation
- Dyspnea
- Swelling of ankles
- Angina pectoris
   a. Fainting (syncope): Spells
                         Seizures
   b. Diabetes.
   c. Hepatitis, jaundice or liver disease.
   d. Tuberculosis.
   e. Sexually transmitted diseases.
   f. Abnormal bleeding associated with previous extraction, surgery and trauma.
   g. Are you allergic to:
- Local anesthesia
- Penicillin or other antibiotics
- Analgesics

- Others:
   – Women:
   – Pregnancy:
   – Nursing:

Habits:
• Clenching	Yes/No
• Mouth breathing	Yes/No
• Tongue thrusting	Yes/No
• Pan-chewing/Tobacco-chewing	Yes/No
• Bruxism	Yes/No
• Chronic lip-biting, cheek-/tongue-biting	Yes/No
• Cigarette- or pipe-smoking	Yes/No

Oral hygiene measures:
1. Age of brush, type of brush.
2. Method of brushing:
   a. Horizontal.
   b. Vertical.
   c. Circular.
3. Frequency of brushing.
4. Estimate of time spent.
5. Interdental aids:
   a. Dental floss, toothpicks.
   b. Interproximal brushes.

OHI–S

16	11	26
46	31	36

16	11	26
46	31	36

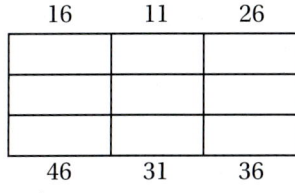

Calculus score: Debris score:
OHI–S score: Interpretation:

Examination
1. **Extraoral examination:**
   a. TMJ: Pain
- Clicking
- Deviation.

b. Symmetry of face.
  c. Lymph nodes—palpable/non-palpable tender/non-tender.
  d. Lip competence.
2. **Intraoral examination**:
   Soft tissue examination:
   a. Buccal and labial mucosa.
   b. Palate.
   c. Floor of the mouth.
   d. Vestibule.
   e. Tongue.

GINGIVAL STATUS

Features	Upper right posterior	Upper anterior	Upper left posterior
Color			
Contour			
Size			
Consistency			
Stippling			
Position			
Bleeding on probing			
Exudation			
Width of attached gingiva			
Features	Lower right posterior	Lower anterior	Lower left posterior
Width of attached gingiva			
Exudation			
Bleeding on probing			
Position			
Stippling			
Consistency			
Size			
Contour			
Color			

Mucogingival problems:

Hard tissue examination:

Number of teeth present:

Missing teeth:

Caries:

Fillings/Restorations:

Impacted teeth:

Hypoplasia/Fluorosis of teeth:

Proximal contact form:

Pathologic migration:

Wasting diseases:
- Attrition:
- Abrasion:
- Erosion:

Tenderness on percussion:

Pulpoperiodontal problems:

Periodontal charting

Teeth	18	17	16	15	14	13	12	11	21	22	23	24	25	26	27	28
Furcation (Glickman's Classification)																
Mobility																
Recession (Miller's Classification)																
Pockets Upper arch (Buccal)																
Lingual																
Lingual																
Pockets Lower arch (Buccal)																
Recession (Miller's Classification)																
Mobility																
Furcation (Glickman's Classification)																
Teeth	48	47	46	45	44	43	42	41	31	32	33	34	35	36	37	38

Occlusal Analysis

- Angle's classification:
- Overjet and overbite:
- Premature contact:
- Crossbite:

Trauma from occlusion:

Fremitus Test: Class I
                Class II
                Class III

Investigations

Radiographic investigations: IOPA radiographs/OPG
- Horizontal bone loss:
- Vertical bone loss:
- Furcation involvement:
- Endotreated/Overhanging restorations:
- Pulpoperiodontal pathology:
- Impacted/Supernumerary/Embedded teeth:
- Caries:

Hematological investigations
Clotting time:
Bleeding time:
RBC:
WBC: Total count:
        Differential count:

Hb%:
Blood sugar analysis: FBS
                         PPBS
                         RBS

Urine examination for: Sugar
                         Albumin
                         Microorganisms

Biopsy:
Bacterial smear:

Provisional diagnosis:

Prognosis:
    Overall:
    Individual:

Treatment plan:
Phase I (etiotropic phase):
Phase II (surgical phase):
Phase III (restorative phase):
Phase IV (maintenance phase):

Case Summary

CHAPTER 2

Recording Clinical Case History

KEY STAGES OF CASE HISTORY RECORDING

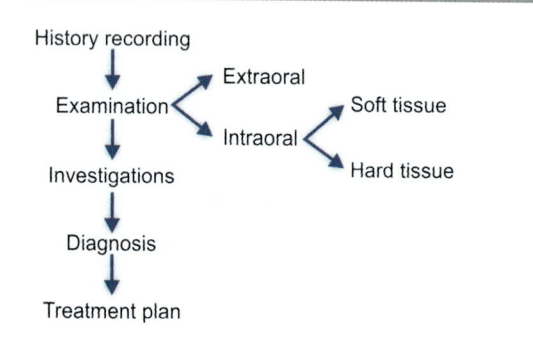

History recording → Examination → Extraoral / Intraoral → Soft tissue / Hard tissue
↓
Investigations
↓
Diagnosis
↓
Treatment plan

HISTORY RECORDING

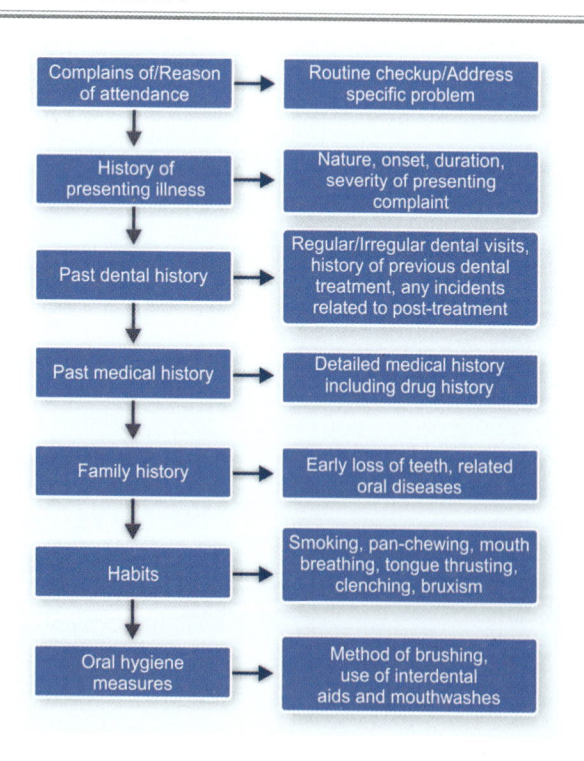

Complains of/Reason of attendance	Routine checkup/Address specific problem
History of presenting illness	Nature, onset, duration, severity of presenting complaint
Past dental history	Regular/Irregular dental visits, history of previous dental treatment, any incidents related to post-treatment
Past medical history	Detailed medical history including drug history
Family history	Early loss of teeth, related oral diseases
Habits	Smoking, pan-chewing, mouth breathing, tongue thrusting, clenching, bruxism
Oral hygiene measures	Method of brushing, use of interdental aids and mouthwashes

CLINICAL EVALUATION, DIAGNOSIS AND TREATMENT PLANNING

Objective

1. A comprehensive periodontal examination not only includes examination of the periodontal status but also complete information regarding the patient's medical history, past dental history, and a thorough soft and hard tissue examination.
2. This will in turn enable the practitioner with a proper diagnosis and treatment plan for the patient.

Patient Interview

This will provide us with chief complaint and previous dental experiences.

Chief Complaint

1. It must be recorded in patient's own words. Many a times patient, when questioned about the purpose of their visit to the dentist, will provide us with his/her desire for a particular treatment. For example:
   - "I want to get a filling done"
   - "I want to clean my teeth"
   - "I want to get my tooth fixed", etc.
2. These should not be recorded as the chief complaint; we need to proceed to ask further questions to derive the chief complaint from the patient, e.g. if a patient says, "I want to get my teeth cleaned", he should be further questioned regarding the reason behind this desire. Then the patient will reveal the actual complaint, i.e. bleeding while brushing.
3. Hence chief complaint sometimes has to be derived from the patient. This is especially true since in periodontitis we deal mostly with chronic problems; the actual problem may be undermined.

Dental History

1. It will provide a picture of both the progress of the current conditions and also the previous efforts of the patient at maintaining their oral health.
2. A history of bleeding gum, change in tooth position, pain, halitosis or a bad taste, oral habits, and previous periodontal care and maintenance may all contribute to a proper diagnosis and determination of prognosis.

Medical History

One has to always remember "never to treat a stranger". A complete medical history must be obtained to:

1. Determine systemic factors or diseases that will require special considerations before, during or after the treatment.
2. A complete list of medications must be obtained in order to identify the drugs or medications that could adversely interact with drugs used in periodontal therapy.

Clinical Examination

Extraoral examination:

1. A complete bimanual and visual examination should be done to uncover unusual growths, lumps or other signs of pathology.
2. A complete muscle and TMJ examination should be done to identify any temporomandibular dysfunction signs and/or symptoms (Figs 2.1 to 2.3).
3. *Examination of lymph nodes:* Since periodontal, periapical and other oral diseases may result in lymph node changes, it is important to examine and evaluate head and neck lymph nodes (Fig. 2.4).

Intraoral examination: A clear understanding of the structure and function of the periodontium is necessary to appreciate the disease process.

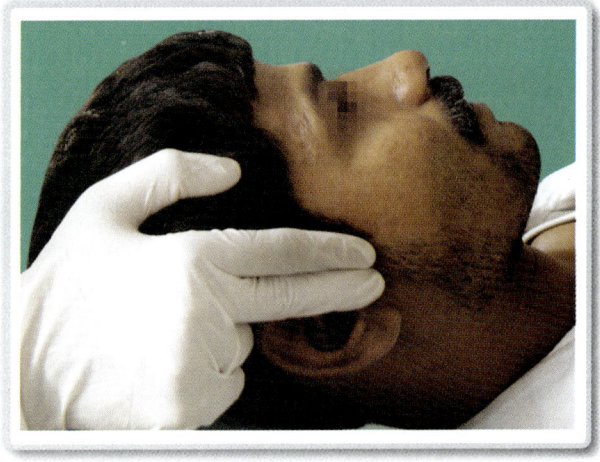

Fig. 2.2: Palpation of the TMJ. Lateral aspect of the joint with mouth closed.

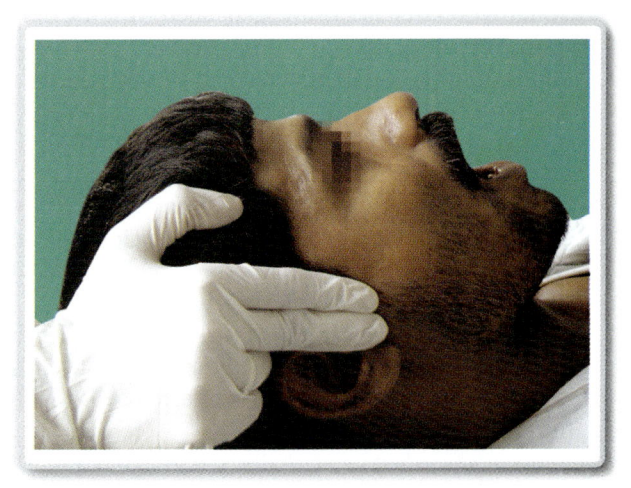

Fig. 2.3: Palpation of the TMJ. Lateral aspect of the joint with mouth open.

Surface Characteristics or Landmarks of the Periodontium (Fig. 2.5)

1. *Free gingiva:* That part of the gingiva that surrounds the tooth and is not directly attached to the tooth surface.

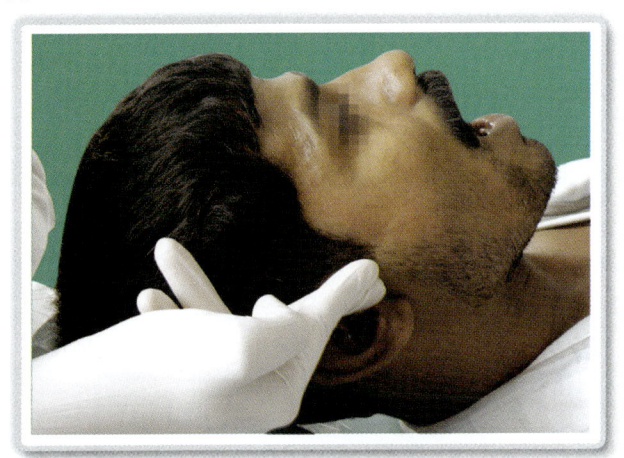

Fig. 2.1: Palpation of the TMJ with the fingers placed behind the condyle

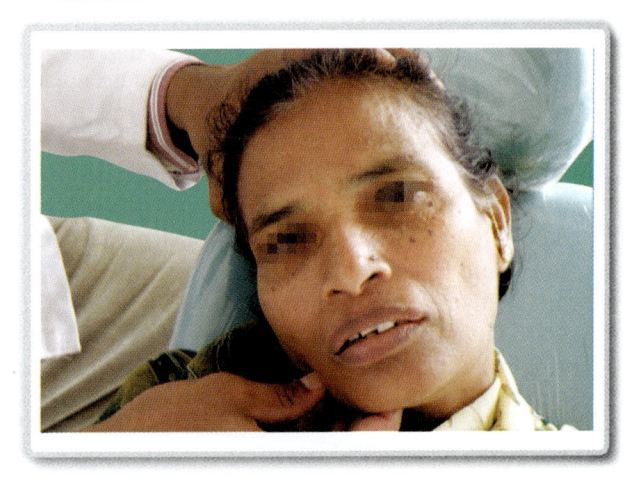

Fig. 2.4: Palpation of the right submandibular lymph node

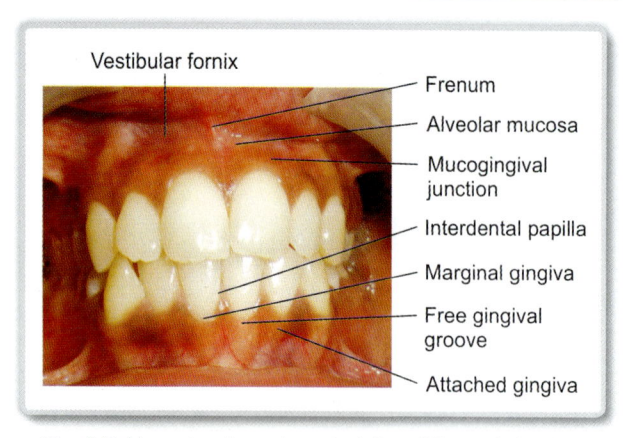

Fig. 2.5: Normal surface characteristics of the periodontium

2. *Free gingival groove:* Shallow V-shaped groove or indentation that is closely associated with the apical extent of free gingiva and runs parallel to the margin of the gingiva. The frequency of its occurrence varies widely.
3. *Attached gingiva:* The portion of the gingiva that is firm, dense, stippled and tightly bound to the underlying periosteum, tooth and bone.
4. *Interdental gingiva/papilla:* That portion of the gingiva that occupies the interproximal spaces. The interdental extension of the gingiva.
5. *Keratinized gingiva:* The surface of the tissue that comprises the marginal and attached gingiva. The epithelium covering this is also referred to as the oral epithelium.
6. *Mucogingival line/junction:* This is the demarcation between the attached gingiva and the alveolar mucosa apical to the attached gingiva.
7. *Alveolar mucosa:* It is the part of the lining mucosa. It is located apical to the attached gingiva. The tissue is loosely attached to the underlying bone, freely movable and relatively fragile.
8. *Frenum/frenulum:* It is a narrow band of tissue that attaches the labial and buccal mucosa to the alveolar mucosa. Lingual frenum is also present.
9. *Rugae:* The irregular ridges in the masticatory mucosa covering the anterior part of the hard palate, adjacent to the incisors, canines and first premolars.
10. *Stippling:* Irregular surface texture similar to the 'orange peel' seen in attached gingiva and central portion of the interdental gingiva.
11. *Sulcus:* It is the space or shallow crevice between the tooth and free gingiva. In health, the sulcus usually measures 1–3 mm depth.
12. *Col:* A valley-like depression of the interdental gingiva that connects facial and lingual papillae and conforms to the shape of the interproximal contact area.

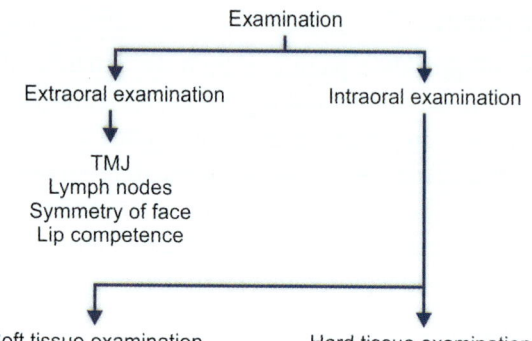

Examination
- Extraoral examination
  - TMJ
  - Lymph nodes
  - Symmetry of face
  - Lip competence
  - Soft tissue examination
    - Buccal and labial mucosa
    - Palate, floor of the mouth
    - Vestibule and tongue
    - Gingival features including color, contour, consistency, surface texture, bleeding on probing
    - Periodontal features including pockets, mucogingival problems
- Intraoral examination
  - Hard tissue examination
    - Missing, carious tooth
    - Restoration, impaction
    - Proximal contact form
    - Furcation involvement, grades I, II, III and IV
    - Mobility, grades I, II and III
    - Pathologic migration
    - Wasting disease
    - Pulpoperiodontal problems
    - Occlusal analysis
    - Trauma from occlusion (fremitus test)

TABLE 2.1: Examination of gingiva in health and disease

Normal color	Changes in the disease with conditions
Coral pink (Fig. 2.6A)	Chronic gingivitis: Varying shades of red, reddish blue, deep blue, pale pink (Fig. 2.6B)
	Acute gingivitis: Bright erythema associated with any pigmentation Gingiva: Black line following the gingival contour, bluish red or deep blue linear pigmentation and violet marginal line
Factors responsible for normal color	Factors responsible for changes in gingival color in disease
Vascular supply	Vascular proliferation (erythematous)
Thickness and degree of keratinization of epithelium	Reduction of keratinization owing to epithelial compression by inflamed tissues (erythematous)
Presence of pigment containing cells	Venous stasis (bluish-red) Perivascular precipitation of metallic sulfides in connective tissue—seen only in inflamed areas due to increased permeability of blood vessels

Contd...

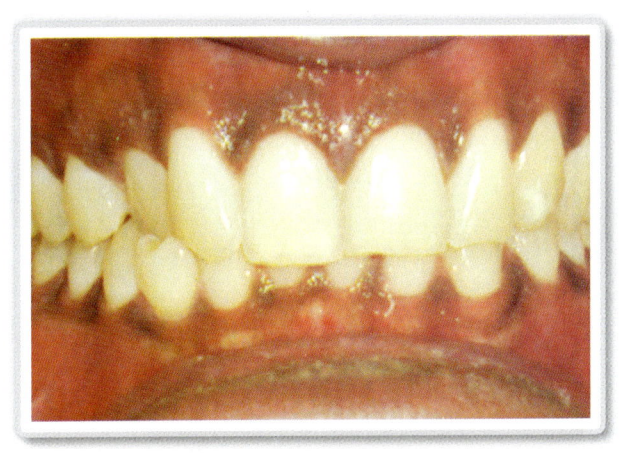

Fig. 2.6A: Color of gingiva in health

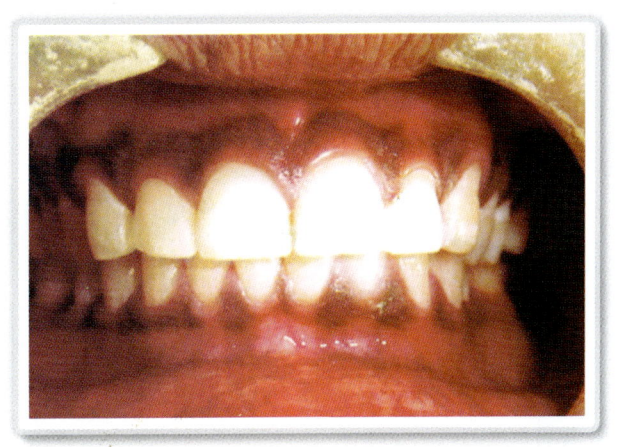

Fig. 2.7A: Contour of the gingiva in health

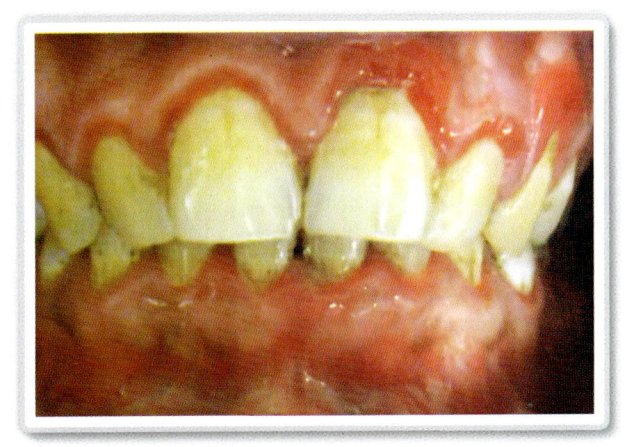

Fig. 2.6B: Erythematous gingiva associated with gingivitis

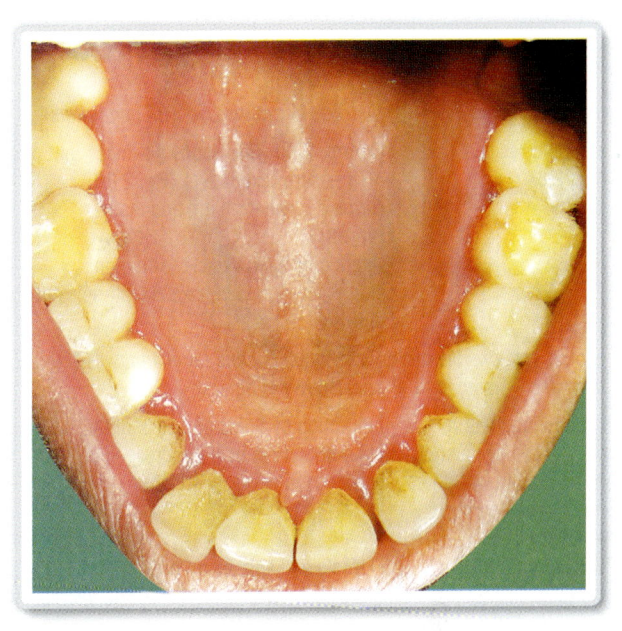

Fig. 2.7B: Gingiva exhibiting rolled margins with blunt papillae

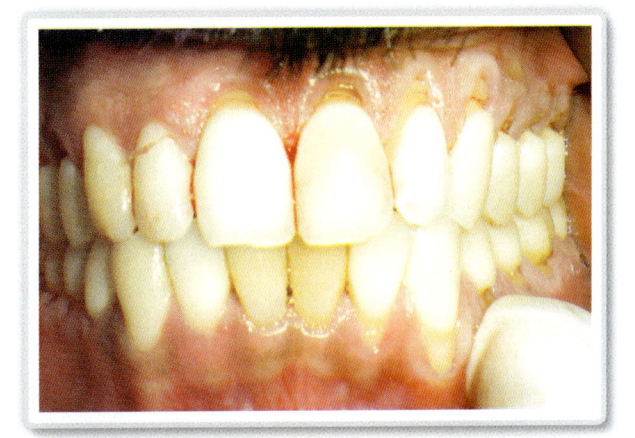

Fig. 2.7C: Exaggerated scalloping

Contd...

Normal contour	*Changes in the disease with conditions*
Marginal gingiva: Scalloped and knife edged	*Chronic gingivitis:* Marginal gingiva becomes rolled and rounded. Interdental papilla becomes blunt and flat
Interdental papilla: Anterior—pyramidal Posterior—tent shaped (Fig. 2.7A)	*Necrotizing ulcerative gingivitis:* Punched out or crater-like depressions at the crest of interdental papilla extending to the marginal gingiva.
	Chronic desquamative gingivitis: Irregularly shaped denuded appearance (Fig. 2.7B)
Factors responsible	*Gingival recession:* Exaggerated scalloping (Fig. 2.7C)
Shape of the tooth and thus the alignment in the arch Location and size of the proximal contact Dimensions of facial and lingual gingival embrasures	*Stillman's cleft:* Apostrophe-shaped indentations extending from and into the gingival margins for varying distances on the facial surfaces (Fig. 2.7D)
	McCall's festoons: Lifesaver-like enlargements of the marginal gingiva

Contd...

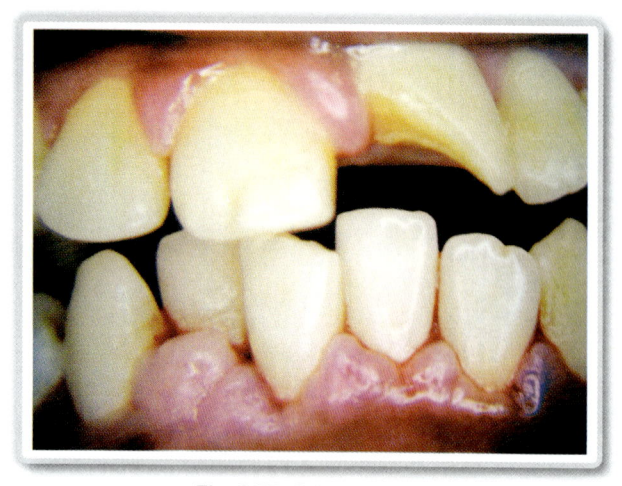

Fig. 2.7D: Stillman's cleft

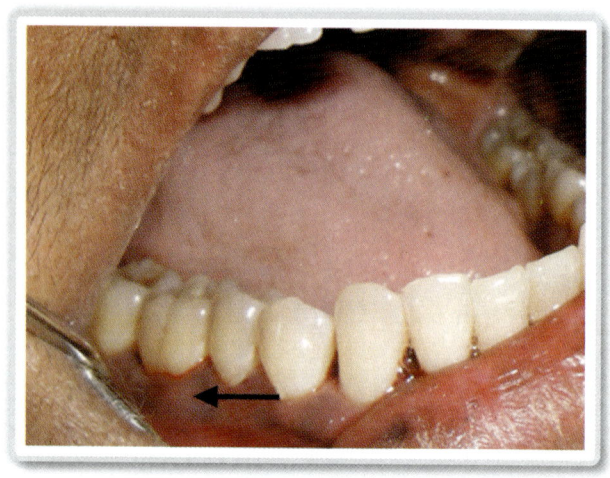

Fig. 2.8B: Pitting on pressure (associated with disease)

Contd...

Normal consistency	Changes in the disease with conditions
Firm and resilient (Fig. 2.8A)	*Chronic gingivitis:* Soggy puffiness that pits on pressure (exudative) (Fig. 2.8B) *Chronic gingivitis:* Firm and leathery (fibrotic) *Acute gingivitis:* Vesicle formation, sloughing—grayish flake like particles of debris
Factors responsible for normal consistency	*Factors responsible for changes in gingival consistency in disease*
Collagenous nature of lamina propria and its contiguity with the mucoperiosteum of alveolar bone Cellular and fluid content of tissue	Infiltration by fluids and cells of the inflammatory exudate (increased cellular content and decreased fibers)—exudative Fibrosis and epithelium proliferation (fibrotic, i.e. increased fibers and decreased inflammatory cells) Intercellular and intracellular edema vesicle formation)

Contd...

Contd...

Normal size	Changes seen in the disease with conditions
Appears normal without any alterations (Fig. 2.9A)	*Gingival enlargement:* The size of the gingiva is enlarged, could be inflammatory or non-inflammatory Mostly associated with pseudo-pockets (Fig. 2.9B)
Factors responsible for normal size of gingiva	*Factors responsible for changes in size during disease*
Sum total of the bulk of cellular and intercellular elements and their vascular supply	Increase in fibers and decrease in cells—non-inflammatory type Increase in cells and decrease in fibers—Inflammatory type Hypertrophy—constitutes an increase in size of cells which results in increase in size of the organ Hyperplasia—constitutes increase in number of cells which results in overall increase in organ size

Contd...

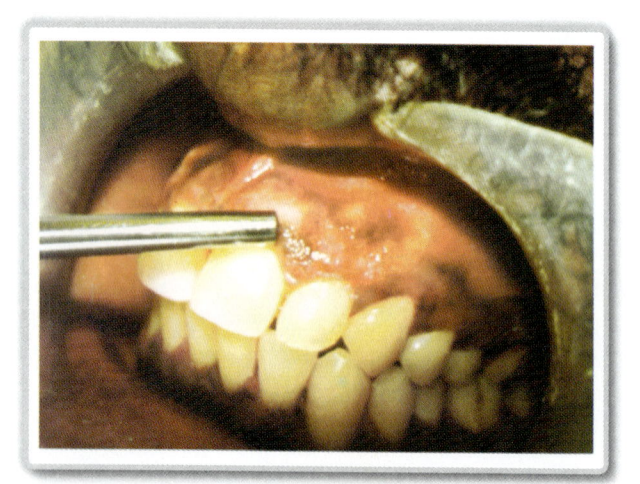

Fig. 2.8A: Normal consistency (blanched appearance)

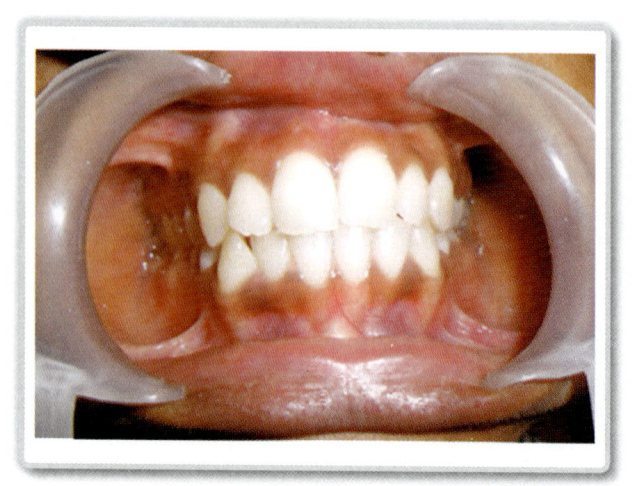

Fig. 2.9A: Normal size of gingiva

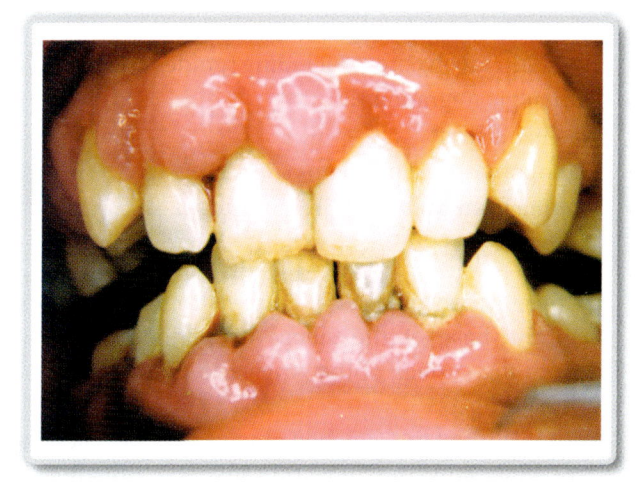

Fig. 2.9B: A case of inflammatory gingival enlargement

Contd...

Normal surface texture	Changes seen in the disease with condition
Stippling (orange peel appearance) is present (viewed by drying) (Fig. 2.10A)	Gingivitis—loss of stippling (Fig. 2.10B) Exudative chronic gingivitis—smooth and shiny Fibrotic chronic gingivitis—firm and nodular Chronic desquamative gingivitis—peeling of the surface Hyperkeratosis—leathery texture Non-inflammatory gingival hyperplasia—minutely nodular surface
Factors responsible for stippling	Factors responsible for the loss of stippling
Due to attachment of the gingival fibers to the underlying bone Microscopically, by alternate rounded protuberance and depressions in the gingival surface	Due to destruction of gingival fibers as a result of inflammation

Contd...

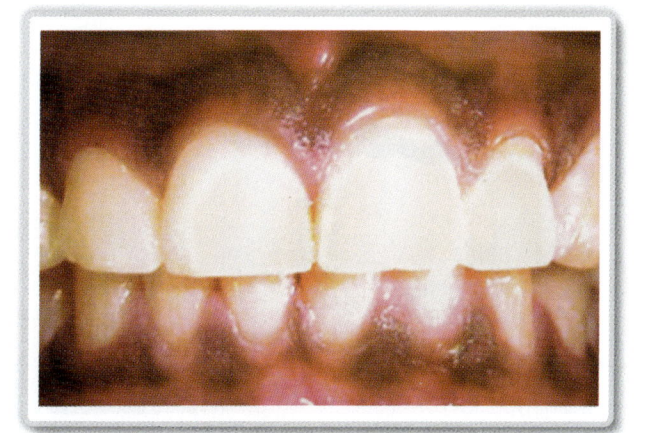

Fig. 2.10A: Normal stippling associated with healthy gingiva

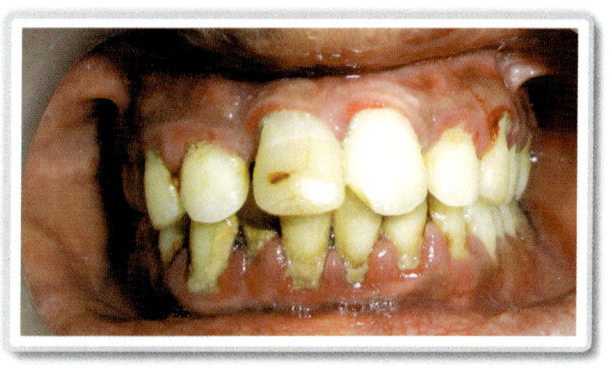

Fig. 2.10B: Absence of stippling in disease

Contd...

Normal position	Changes in the disease with condition
Is 1 millimeter above the cementoenamel junction (CEJ) (Fig. 2.11A)	Apically shifted—gingival recession (Fig. 2.11B) Coronally shifted—pseudopockets (Fig. 2.11C)
Factors responsible for normal position	Factors responsible for change in gingival position in disease
Position of the tooth in the arch Root bone angle Mesiodistal curvature	Toothbrush trauma Gingival inflammation High frenum attachment Tooth malposition Friction from soft tissues (gingival ablation)

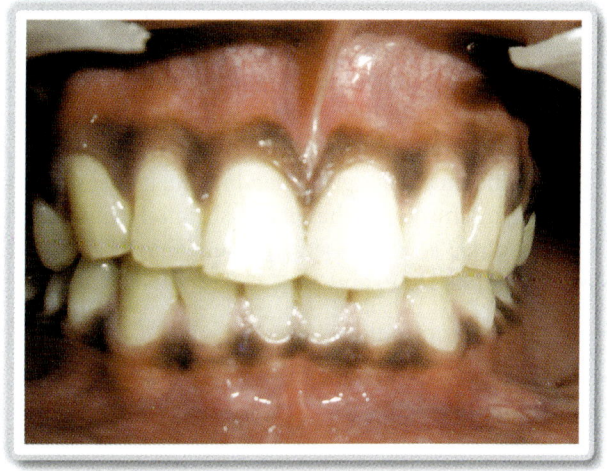

Fig. 2.11A: Position of the marginal gingiva in health

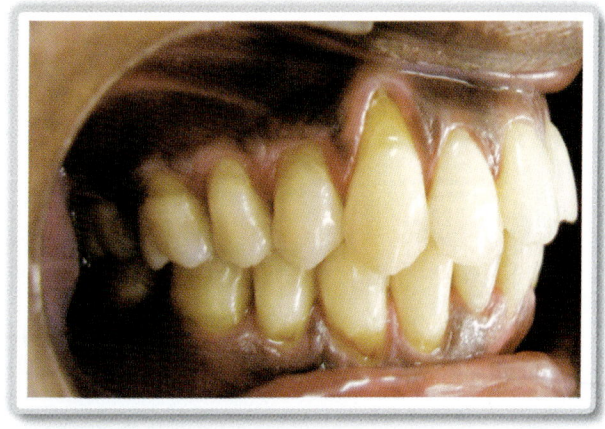

Fig. 2.11B: Changes seen in the position of the gingiva in disease (gingival recession)

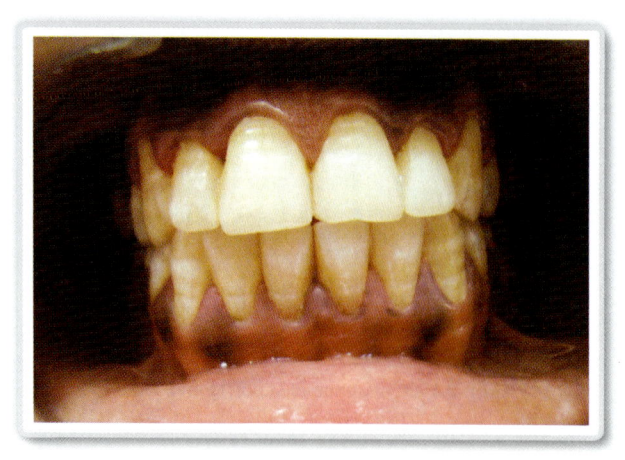

Fig. 2.11C: Coronal migration of marginal gingiva (pseudopocket) in upper anteriors

Bleeding on Probing (Fig. 2.12)

Normally, gingival bleeding is not evident. In disease:
1. Bleeding may occur spontaneously or delayed by 30–60 seconds. It can be checked by using a blunt periodontal probe. Bleeding is still the most reliable indicator of the presence of gingival or periodontal inflammation.
2. The amount of bleeding and the amount of time between stimulation and the appearance of blood can be used to judge the severity of inflammation, i.e. spontaneous bleeding more severe the inflammation.
3. Bleeding scores may be calculated as a percentage of sites around a tooth that bleeds or that do not bleed.
4. Significance of gingival bleeding, factors responsible and microscopic changes associated with gingival bleeding is discussed in detail in Chapter 53, Questions 18, 19 and 20.

Hard Tissue Examination
- Missing carious teeth
- Restoration
- Proximal contact form
- Furcation involvement including (grades I, II, III, IV)
- Pathologic migration
- Wasting disease
- Pulpoperiodontal problems
- Trauma from occlusion (fremitus test).

Amount of Attached Gingiva

1. The attached gingiva is measured from the projection of the base of the sulcus or periodontal pocket onto the surface of the gingiva to the mucogingival junction.
2. The width of the attached gingiva may be calculated by subtracting the sulcus/pocket depth from the total width of the gingiva, i.e. from the free gingival margin to the mucogingival junction (Fig. 2.13).
    Width of attached gingiva =
    Total gingival width – Pocket depth.
3. Width of attached gingiva is adequate or not can be determined by four different methods (refer Chapter 53, Question 22):
    a. Measurement approach.
    b. Using Schiller's potassium iodide solution.
    c. Tension test.
    d. Roll test.

    To summarize, the gingival examination should be done in a systematic manner and any changes in the gingival features (color, contour, consistency, size and others) can directly influence the diagnosis of the case.
4. Always record these findings according to the arch, sextant and surface of the tooth (i.e. upper right posteriors, labial/palatal/lingual surfaces).
5. Follow the gingival status format provided in the case history proforma, which will help us not to miss any important gingival findings.

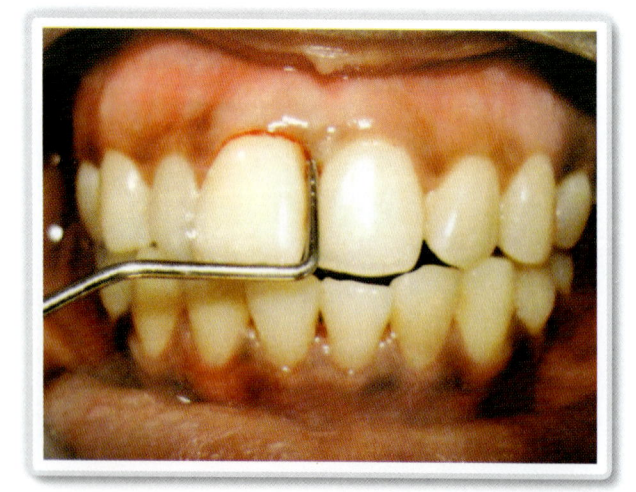

Fig. 2.12: Clinical demonstration of bleeding on probing

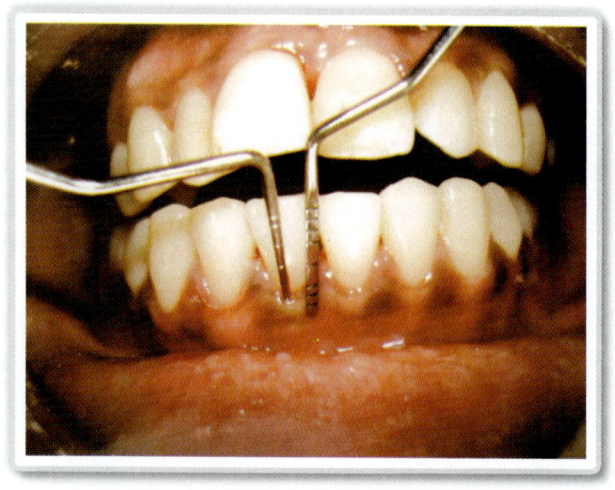

Fig. 2.13: Determination of width of attached gingiva

CHAPTER 2 Recording Clinical Case History

Periodontal Examination

- Periodontal pocket probing
- Attachment level measurements
- Furcation examination
- Mobility
- Fremitus test.

Periodontal Pocket Probing

There are two different types of pocket depths:
- The biologic or histologic depth
- The clinical or probing depth.

The probing depth measurement is recorded from the gingival margin to the base of the pocket.

Technique of Probing for the Identification of Pockets

1. The depth of the periodontal pocket is measured by using a calibrated periodontal probe.
2. The probe is inserted along the long axis of the tooth into the pocket with gentle force (approximately 25 g) until resistance is met (Fig. 2.14A).
3. Force of 25 g is necessary to indent the pad of thumb about 1–2 mm (Fig. 2.14B).
4. The probe is walked around each surface of the tooth (Fig. 2.14C).
5. Each tooth is examined at six locations, i.e. the mesiobuccal, buccal, distobuccal, distolingual, lingual, mesiolingual (Fig. 2.14D).
6. Mostly the probe is held parallel to the long axis of the tooth and 'walked' circumferentially around each surface of the tooth.
7. In interproximal surfaces to detect the craters the probe may have to be angled obliquely or 10° on each buccal and lingual surfaces.

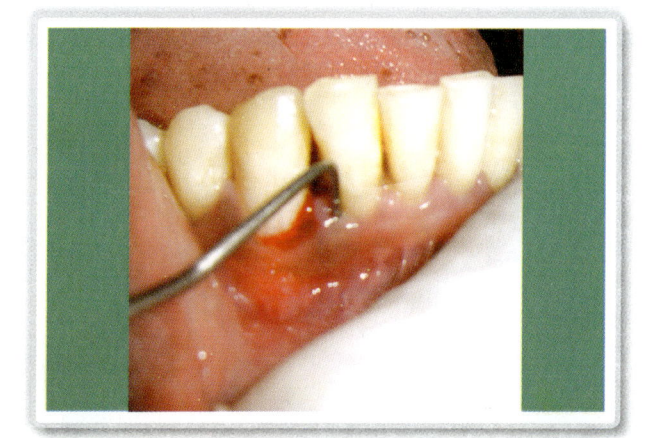

Fig. 2.14A: Probing technique (probe held parallel to the long axis of tooth)

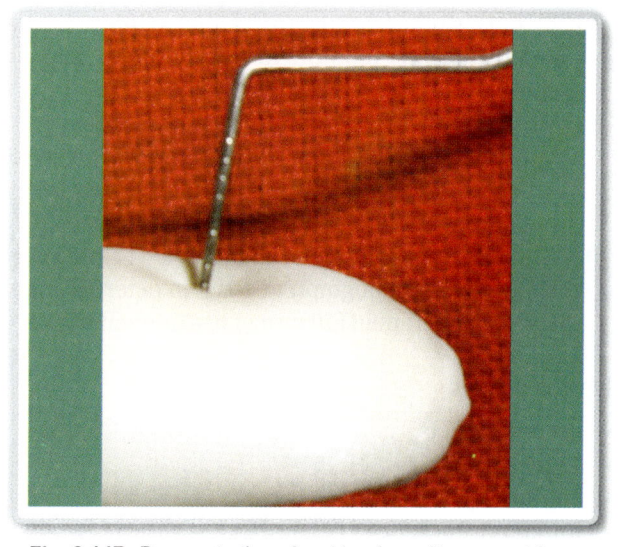

Fig. 2.14B: Demonstration of probing force (the correct force depresses the thumb pad 1–2 mm)

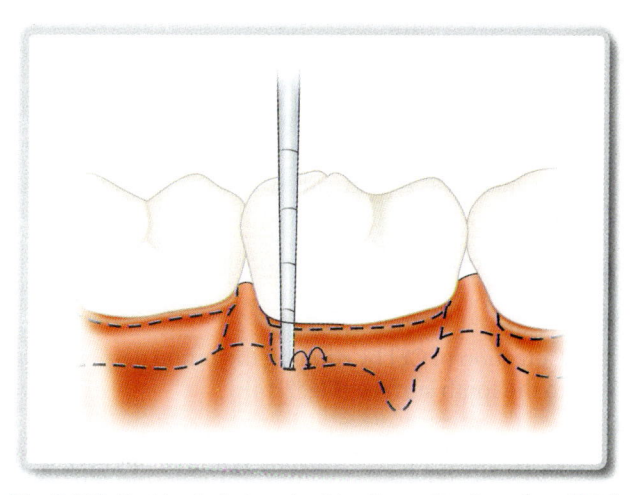

Fig. 2.14C: Probing technique (walking the probe circumferentially)

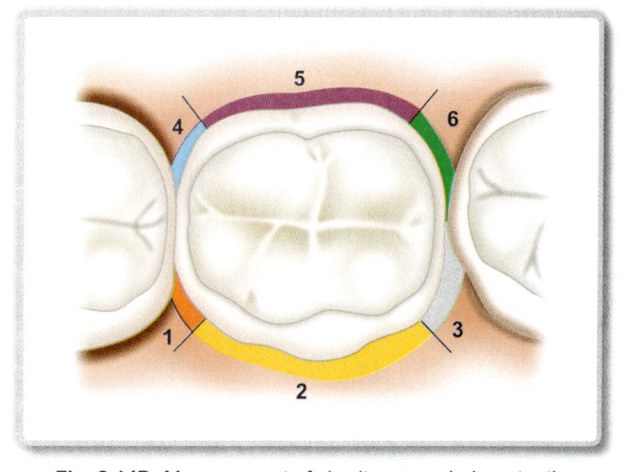

Fig. 2.14D: Measurement of six sites recorded per tooth

8. Various studies have proved that clinical probing depth is greater than the histologic sulcus or pocket depth.
9. Most importantly, pockets are not detected by radiologic examination because pocket is a soft tissue change. Only bone loss can be detected by radiographs where pockets may be suspected.
10. Gutta-percha points or calibrated silver points can be used with radiograph to assist in determining the level of attachment (10 mm of periodontal pocket).

Types of Pockets

- Pseudopockets
- True pockets
- Suprabony pockets
- Infrabony pockets.

Measurement of True Pockets
(Refer Chapter 53, Question 24)

1. True pockets are associated with apical migration of junctional epithelium (attachment loss).
2. Normally, junctional epithelium is attached at the cementoenamel junction (CEJ), hence CEJ is considered as a landmark for determining attachment loss.

How do You Detect a True Pocket?

Step 1

1. Detection of CEJ by running the probe perpendicular to the tooth surface (Fig. 2.14E).

Step 2

1. Once the CEJ is detected, without dislodging the probe, bring it back to parallel position and observe whether the probing can be done beyond this point. If it can, then it is understood that the junctional epithelium is shifted apically—a true pocket (Fig. 2.14F).

True pockets can never be diagnosed based on the enormity of depth of the pocket. For example, the deeper pocket—more attachment loss, is the wrong notion that many students perceive.

Presence of gingival enlargement should not be considered solely for the diagnosis of the pseudopockets because there could also be a combined pocket wherein we see both gingival enlargement and attachment loss.

Hence proper probing steps has to be followed for detection of true pockets.

Suprabony Pockets (Fig. 2.14G)

It is a true pocket with the base of pocket coronal to underlying alveolar bone crest. Clinically, it can be assessed by probing measurements. After the probe is inserted into the gingival sulcus, when lateral pressure is applied, if soft tissue resistance is felt, then it can be diagnosed as a suprabony pocket. This is based on the fact that suprabony pockets are associated with horizontal bone loss. Hence there is no bony resistance felt because all the walls of the alveolar crest are lost in the horizontal bone loss.

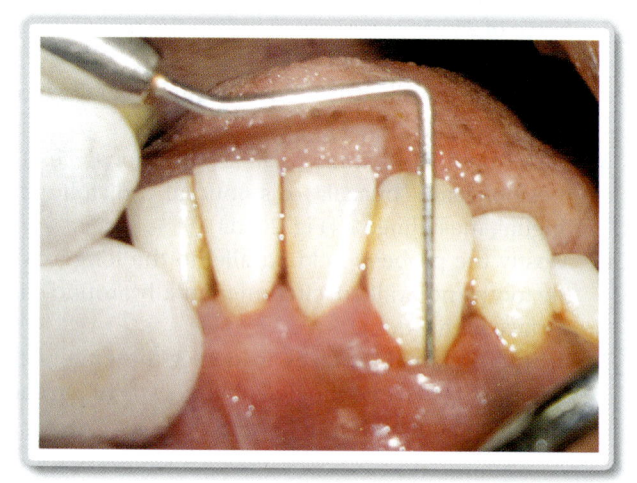

Fig. 2.14F: Probe being brought back to parallel position to check for attachment loss

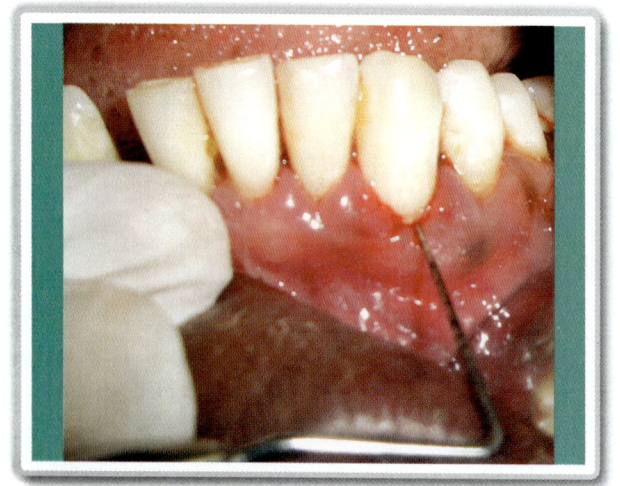

Fig. 2.14E: Detection of CEJ (probe in perpendicular position)

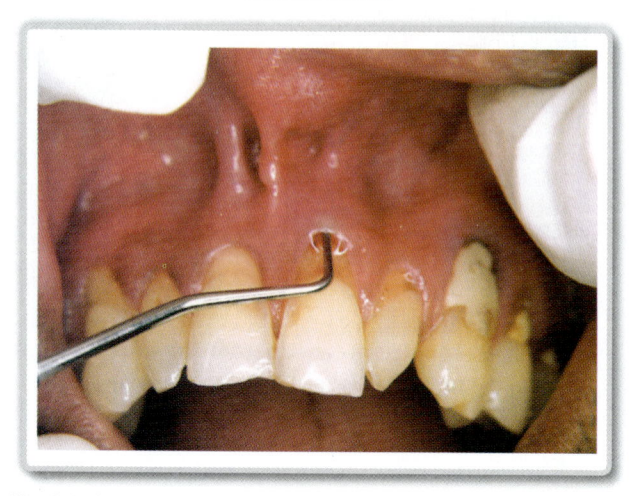

Fig. 2.14G: Suprabony/Infrabony pocket (probe in place with lateral pressure)

Infrabony Pockets

It has the base of the pocket apical to the crest of alveolar bone and is associated with vertical bone loss. Hence on probing with lateral pressure hard tissue resistance is felt because part of bony crest may be present.

Determination of the Level of Attachment (Figs 2.15A to C)

1. Pocket depth is the distance between the base of the pocket and the crest of gingival margin whereas the level of attachment is the distance between the base of the pocket and fixed reference point on the crown, such as CEJ.
2. Attachment level can be determined based on the location of gingival margin.

Situation I	Situation II	Situation III
When the gingival margin coincides with the CEJ, the loss of attachment equals the pocket depth. Attachment loss = pocket depth	When the gingival margin is located apical to the CEJ. Distance between the CEJ and gingival margin (GM) is added to the pocket depth	When the gingival margin is located on the anatomic crown. Distance between the CEJ and gingival margin (GM) is subtracted from the pocket depth

Sample Periodontal Chart (Fig. 2.16)

Furcation Examination

1. The furcation, the anatomic area of a multirooted tooth where the roots diverge, may be examined with a furcation probe such as the Nabers probe. Even an explorer can be used to detect the furcation.
2. Furcations are probed by placing the tip of the Nabers probe against the tooth and moving it in apical direction. The depression of the furcation can be felt in this manner (Figs 2.17A and B):
   a. Maxillary premolars: Mesial furcation to be examined.
   b. Maxillary molars: Buccal, mesial and distal furcas to be examined.
   c. Mandibular molars: Buccal, lingual furcas to be examined.

The mesial furcation of maxillary first and second molars must be approached from the palate due to the shape of the mesial and palatal roots.

Tooth A
When the gingival margin is located at the CEJ →
Attachement loss = Probing depth (6 mm)
AL = 6 mm

Tooth B
When the gingival margin is located apical to the CEJ →
Attachment loss = Probing depth (3 mm) + Distance from CEJ to gingival margin (3 mm)
AL = 3 mm + 3 mm
  = 6 mm

Tooth C
When the gingival margin is located on the anatomic crown
Attachment Loss = Probing depth (9 mm) − Distance from CEJ to gingival margin (3 mm)
AL = 9 mm − 3 mm
   = 6 mm

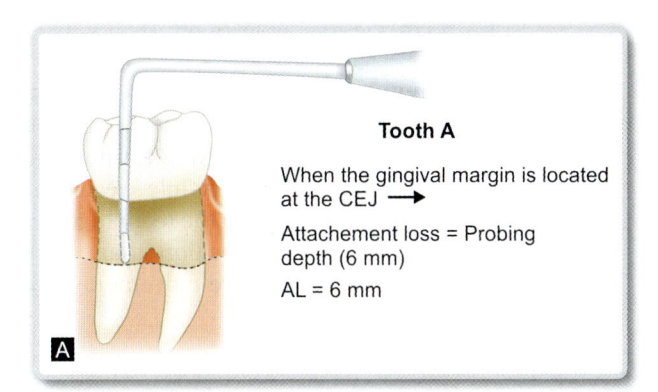

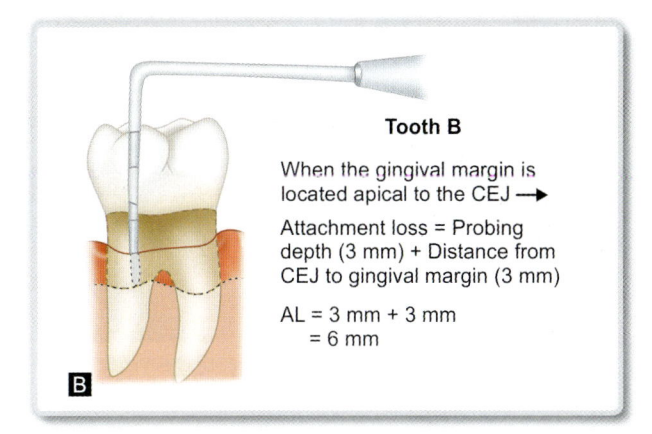

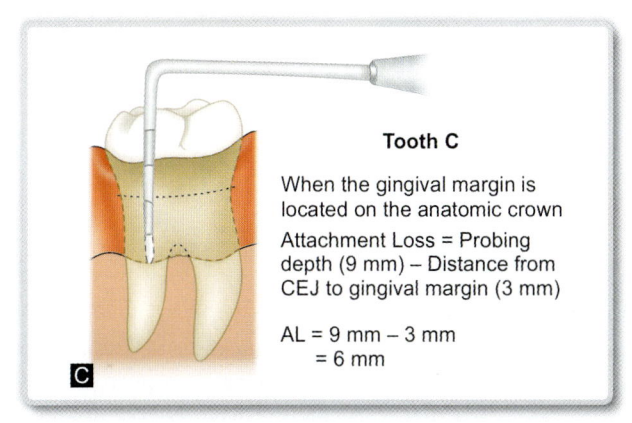

Figs 2.15A to C: Determination of the level of attachment

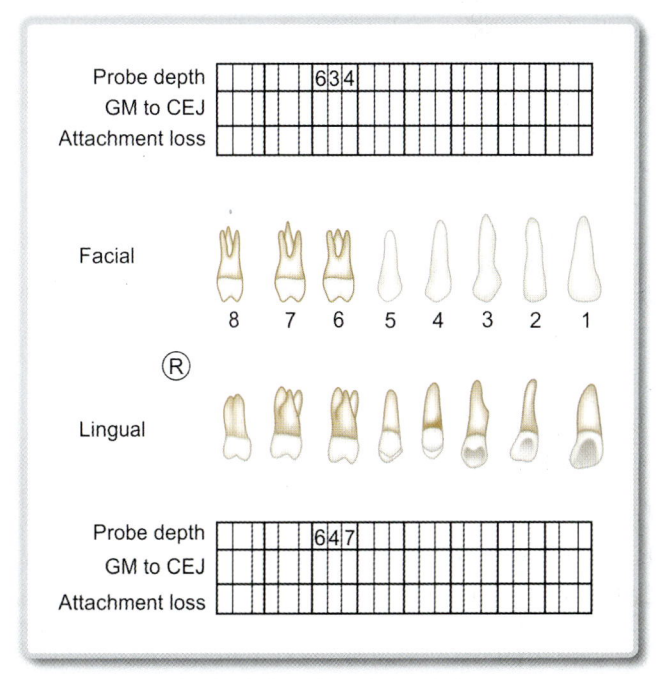

Fig. 2.16: Sample periodontal chart

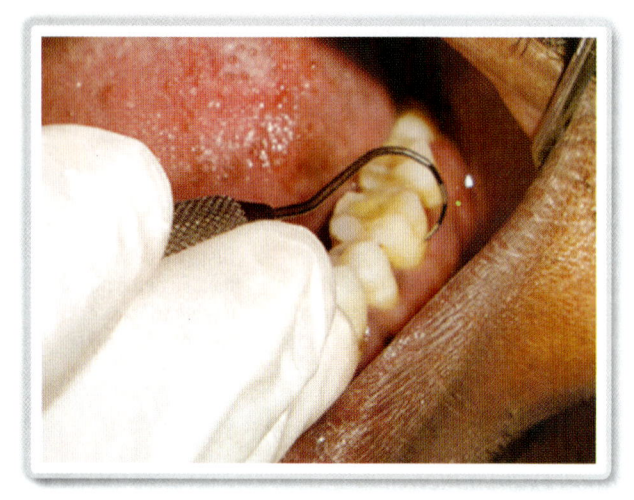

Fig. 2.17A: Detection of furcation entrance

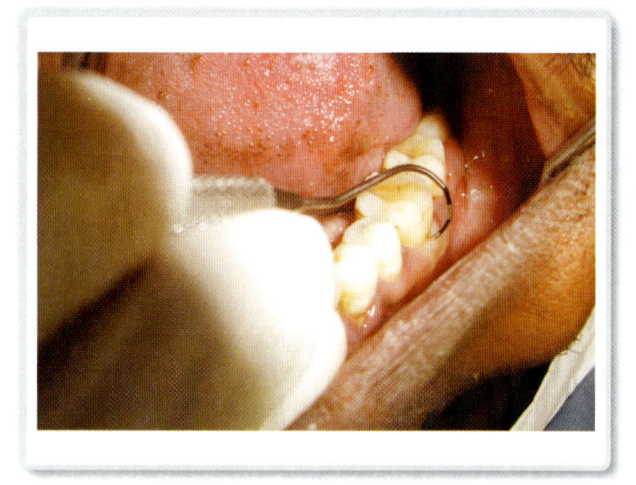

Fig. 2.17B: Furcation examination

Glickman's Furcation Classification

Grade I: Incipient bone loss. The furcation probe can feel the depression of the furcation opening.

Grade II: Partial bone loss (cul-de-sac). The furcation probe tip enters partially under the roof of the furcation.

Grade III: Total bone loss with through-and-through opening of the furcation. The furcation entrance is not visible.

Grade IV: A grade III furcation where the furcation entrance is visible.

Various other classifications of furcation involvement are provided in Chapter 53, Question 29.

Mobility

It is defined as the movement of a tooth in the socket as a result of externally applied force:
1. Mobility is measured by the examiner pushing the tooth gently in a faciolingual direction using the blunt ends of a two metal instruments, usually a mirror handle and handle of a periodontal probe (Fig. 2.18).
2. Mobility may be recorded on 0–3 scale:
   0: No mobility
   1: Mobility that is perceptible
   2: Mobility < 1 mm faciolingually, but no apical movement
   3: Apical movement as well as lateral movement > 1 mm.

   Other classifications of mobility are discussed in detail in Chapter 5.

Fremitus

It is a palpable or visible movement of a tooth when subjected to occlusal forces:
1. Fremitus may be detected both in centric occlusion and in lateral excursive movements (lateral fremitus) (Fig. 2.19).
2. To measure fremitus, dampened index finger (wet finger can perceive the vibrations better) is placed on the tooth in question or by looking as the teeth come together or are moved. While recording fremitus the patient is asked to tap the teeth together in the maximum intercuspal position then grind systematically in lateral, protrusive movements and positions.

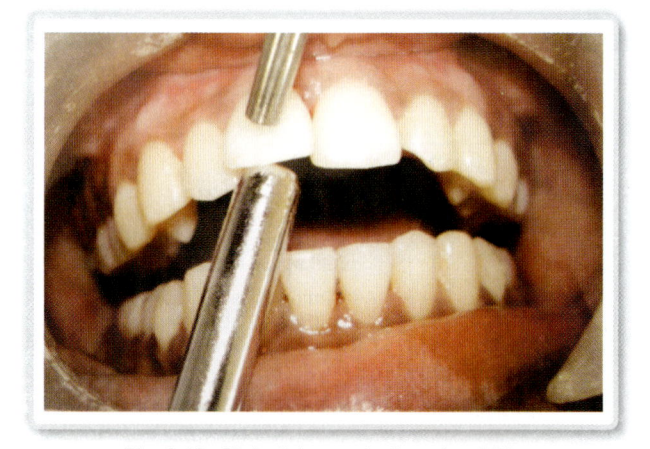

Fig. 2.18: Clinical demonstration of mobility

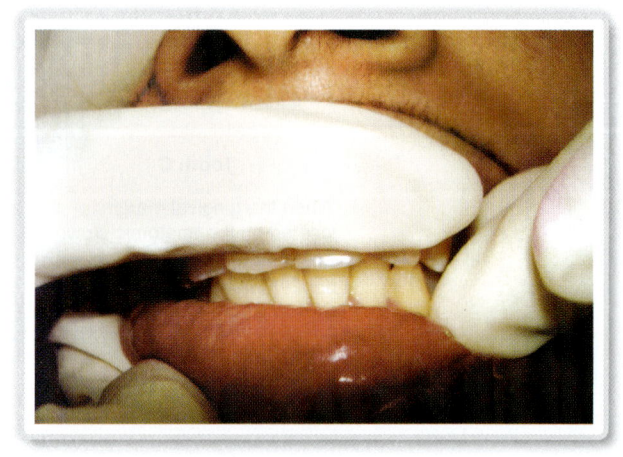

Fig. 2.19: Clinical demonstration of fremitus

3. Fremitus is recorded as:
   a. Class I fremitus: Mild vibration and movements detected.
   b. Class II fremitus: Easily palpable vibration, but no visible movements.
   c. Class III fremitus: Movements visible with naked eye.

INVESTIGATIONS

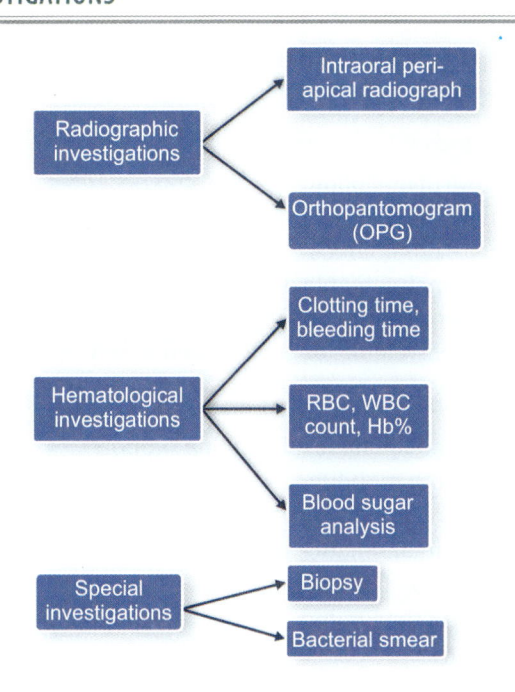

- Soft tissue changes such as color, bleeding on probing, etc.
- Amount of plaque and calculus (relevant in aggressive periodontitis cases)

```
Radiographic investigations → Intraoral peri-apical radiograph
                            → Orthopantomogram (OPG)

Hematological investigations → Clotting time, bleeding time
                             → RBC, WBC count, Hb%
                             → Blood sugar analysis

Special investigations → Biopsy
                      → Bacterial smear
```

```
Diagnosis
├── Clinical features
│   • Bleeding on probing
│   • Change in color of gingival
│   • Periodontal probing depth of 3 mm or less
│   • Bone loss (crestal)
│   → Gingivitis; either acute or chronic
│       → Localized / Generalized
│
└── Clinical features
    • Periodontal probing more than 3 mm and attachment loss
    • Furcation involvement
    • Bleeding on probing
    • Recession
    • Bone loss more than ⅓rd of root length
    • Mobility
    → Periodontitis Chronic/Aggressive
```

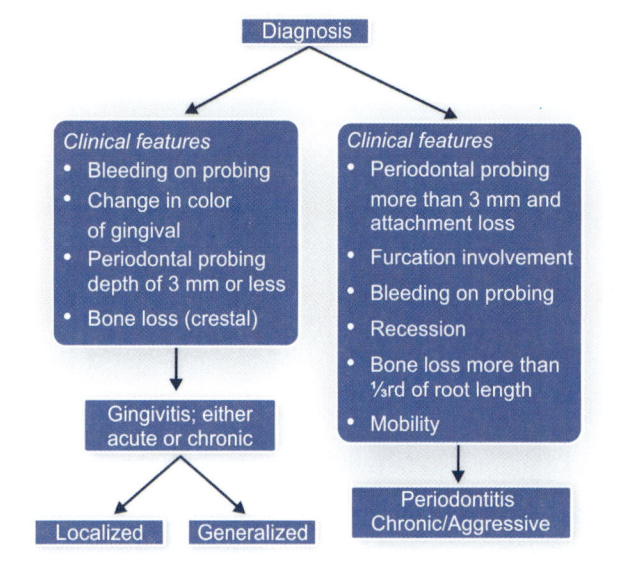

- Pocket depth
- Attachment loss, patterns of attachment loss (difference in clinical picture and radiographic findings)
- Mobility
- Furcation involvement, etc.
- Progression of disease
- Involvement of dentition (localized and generalized)
- Diagnostic aids (if available)
  - IOPA/OPG
  - GCF markers.

Diagnosis

After proper case history recording, the diagnosis of periodontal disease is based on the interpretation of various clinical findings.

Key Points to Note Before Arriving at a Diagnosis

- Age of patient/Geographic location of the patient
- Chief complaint of patient
- Medical history; for instance as it is important in aggressive periodontitis cases
- Familial history (as in cases of aggressive periodontitis)

PROGNOSIS

The term prognosis has been used to indicate the prediction of the future course of a distance in terms of disease outcomes following its onset and/or treatment.

Kornman and colleagues in 2000 noted that we must not confuse risk potential by basing future prognosis on the current diagnostic assessment, "For unlike diagnosis that looks at what it is, prognosis determines what may become of the disease".

Periodontitis

Chronic:
- Slight (1–2 mm)
- Moderate (3–4 mm)
- Severe (≥ 5 mm)

Aggressive: Localized / Generalized

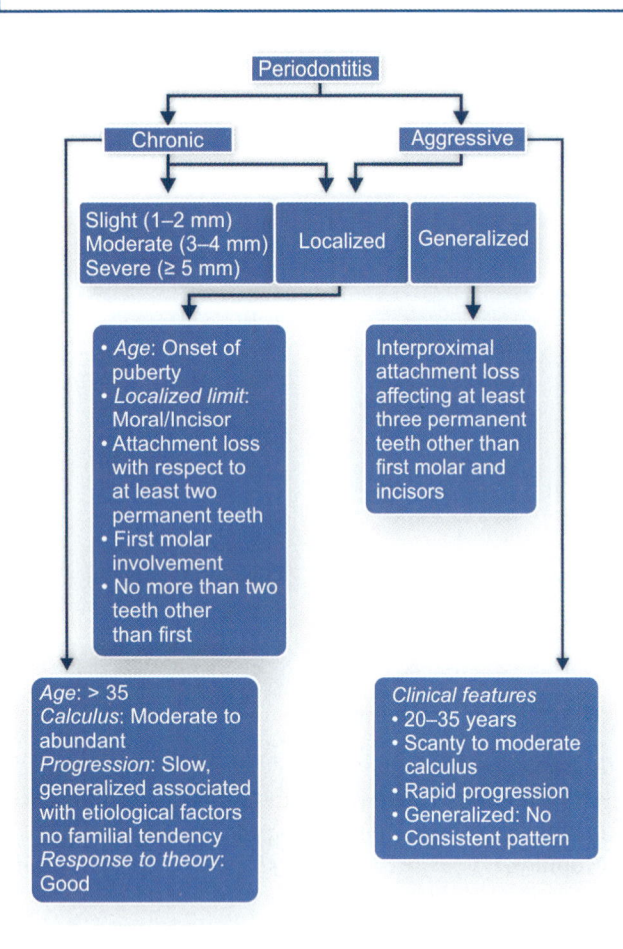

Localized:
- *Age*: Onset of puberty
- *Localized limit*: Moral/Incisor
- Attachment loss with respect to at least two permanent teeth
- First molar involvement
- No more than two teeth other than first

Generalized:
- Interproximal attachment loss affecting at least three permanent teeth other than first molar and incisors

Chronic details:
- *Age*: > 35
- *Calculus*: Moderate to abundant
- *Progression*: Slow, generalized associated with etiological factors no familial tendency
- *Response to theory*: Good

Generalized clinical features:
- 20–35 years
- Scanty to moderate calculus
- Rapid progression
- Generalized: No
- Consistent pattern

CLINICAL FACTORS USED IN DETERMINING PROGNOSIS

Individual Prognosis
- Percentage of bone loss
- Deepest probing depth
- Horizontal or vertical bone loss
- Deepest furcation involvement: 1, 2, 3
- Mobility: 0, 1, 2, 3
- Crown to root ratio: Favorable/Unfavorable
- Caries or pulpal involvement: Yes/No
- Tooth malposition: Yes/No
- Fixed or removable abutment: Yes/No.

Overall Prognosis
- Age
- Significant medical history (smoker or non-smoker)
- Family history of periodontal disease (mother, father or sibling): Yes/No and whom
- Hygiene: Good, fair, poor
- Complaint: Yes/No
- Maintenance intervals: 2 months, 2 months alternate, 3 months and 3 months alternate
- Parafunctional habit with bite guard
- Parafunctional habit without bite guard.

Types of Prognosis

Careful analyzing of these factors allows clinician to establish one of the following prognosis.

Excellent Prognosis
- No bone loss
- Excellent gingival condition
- Good patient cooperation
- No systemic or environmental factors.

Good Prognosis

One or more of the following:
- Adequate remaining bone support
- Adequate possibilities to control etiological factors and establish maintainable dentition
- Patient cooperation positive
- Absence of systemic or environmental factors.

Fair Prognosis
- Less than adequate residual bone support
- Grade I tooth mobility
- Grade I furcation involvement
- Adequate maintenance possible
- Acceptable patient cooperation
- Presence of the limited systemic and/or environmental factors.

Poor Prognosis
- Moderate to advanced bone loss
- Tooth mobility
- Grade I and II furcation involvements
- Difficult-to-maintain areas
- Doubtful patient compliance
- Presence of systemic/environmental factors.

Questionable Prognosis
- Advanced bone loss
- Grade II and III furcation involvements
- Tooth mobility
- Inaccessible areas
- Presence of systemic/environmental factors.

Hopeless Prognosis
- Advanced bone loss
- Non-maintainable areas
- Extractions indicated
- Presence of the uncontrolled systemic/environmental factors.

Periodontal Prognosis Checklist

Factors	Favorable	Unfavorable
Smoking		
Non-smoker	√	
Heavy smoker		√
Parafunction		
With night guard	√	
Without night guard		√
Motivation/Cooperation		
Low plaque	√	
High plaque		√
Unfavorable systemic factors		√

Tooth and site anatomic factors	Favorable	Unfavorable
Mobility		
None	√	
Grade I	√	
Grade II		√
Grade III		√
Note: Loose teeth do not make for good long-term prognosis		
Initial probing depth		
0–3 mm	√	
4–6 mm	√–?	
7–10 mm		√
Note: More the probing depth less favorable is the prognosis. Increased probing depth is a very negative prognosticator		
Initial bone level (IBL)		
0%–25%	√	
25%–50%	√–?	
50%		√
Note: IBL is greater prognosticator than residual bone level		
Crown to root ratio		
1:2–1:5	√	
1:1.5–1	√	
1:1		√
Bone topography (amenable to GTR)		
Horizontal bone loss		√
Infrabony defect (2–3 walls)	√	

Contd...

Contd...

	Favorable	Unfavorable
Hemiseptum (1 wall) Deeper the intrabony defects better is the prognosis		√
Furcation		
No involvement	√	
Grade I	√	
Grade II (early)	√	
Deep grade II and III		√
Occlusion		
Stable	√	
Unstable		
• Missing teeth posterior collapse		√
• No incisal guidance		√
• Progressive tooth mobility (PTM)		√
• Crowding		√
• Wear facets		√
Bruxism		√
Clenching		
• Primary trauma	√	
• Secondary trauma		√

Note: If primary occlusal trauma cannot be adequately corrected to reduce mobility, the tooth should be considered questionable

PERIODONTAL TREATMENT PLAN

Periodontal diagnosis and treatment planning are critical steps in the process of periodontal disease management. Diagnosis and treatment planning are the direct outcomes of a periodontal assessment (Figs 2.20 and 2.21).

An accurate treatment plan should be based upon a comprehensive assessment of periodontal signs and patient symptoms.

While all periodontal treatment plans share a common goal (i.e. control of inflammatory periodontal diseases), the pathway to that goal from patient to patient is rarely the same.

The factors that decide the individual periodontal therapy are:
- Patient's own desire
- Patient's age
- Financial circumstances
- Preference of individual clinician.

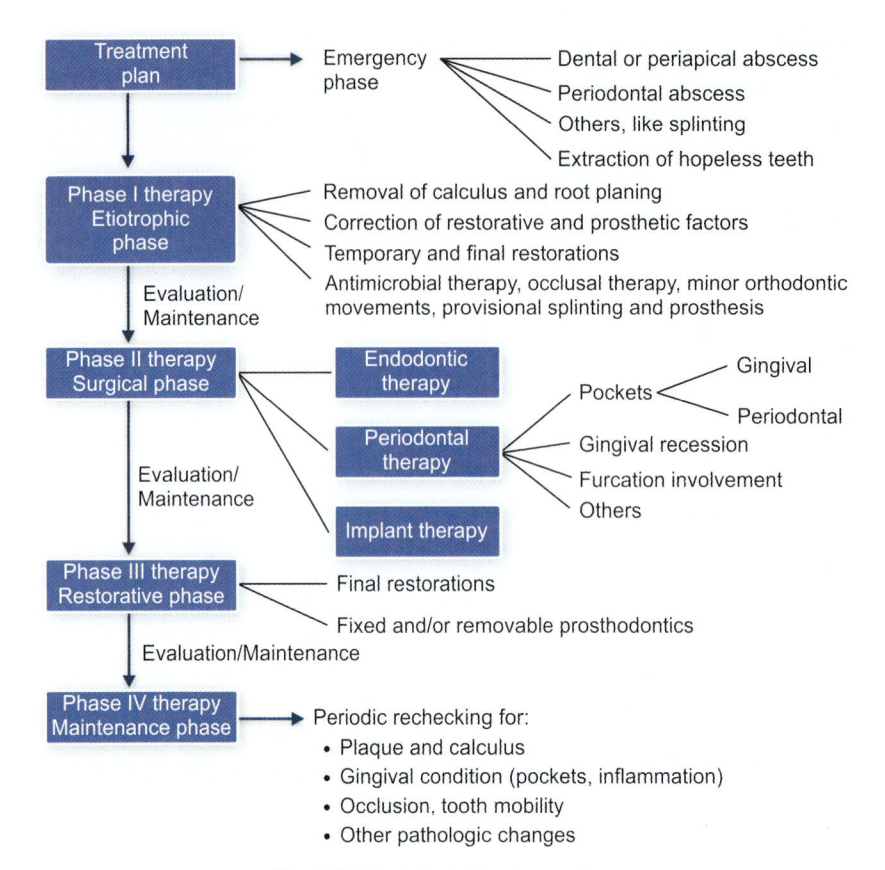

Fig. 2.20: Periodontal treatment plan

TREATMENT OF GINGIVITIS

After proper diagnosis is made the treatment sequencing in gingivitis is as follows.

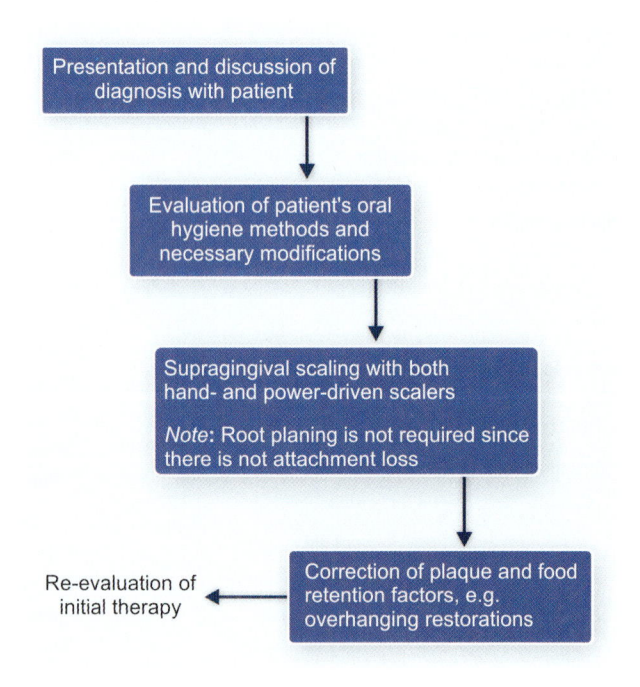

Fig. 2.21: Periodontal treatment plan (continued)

CHRONIC PERIODONTITIS

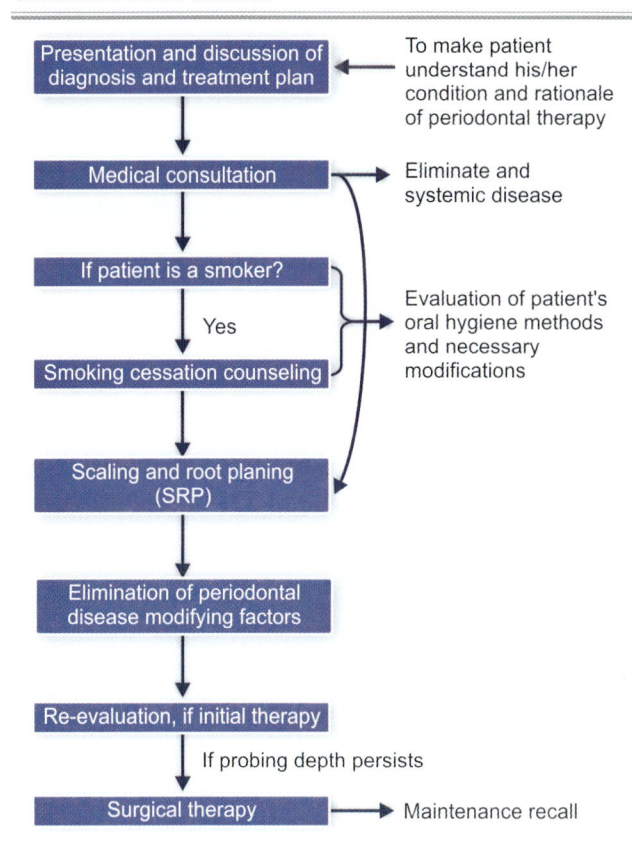

```
Presentation and discussion of   ←  To make patient
diagnosis and treatment plan         understand his/her
            ↓                        condition and rationale
                                     of periodontal therapy
      Medical consultation       →  Eliminate and
            ↓                        systemic disease
    If patient is a smoker?
            ↓ Yes                    Evaluation of patient's
  Smoking cessation counseling       oral hygiene methods
            ↓                        and necessary
                                     modifications
   Scaling and root planing
            (SRP)
            ↓
    Elimination of periodontal
    disease modifying factors
            ↓
   Re-evaluation, if initial therapy
            ↓ If probing depth persists
      Surgical therapy           →  Maintenance recall
```

TISSUE RESPONSE TO PERIODONTAL THERAPY

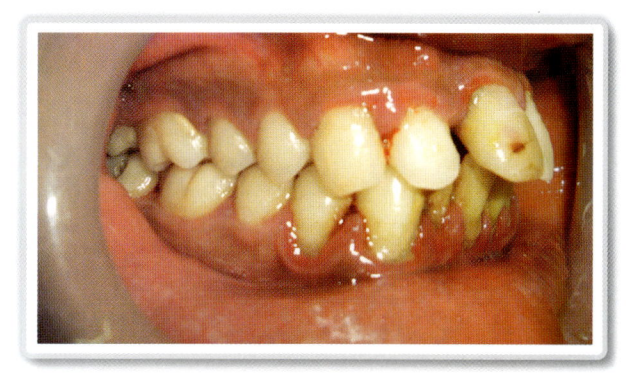

Case 1
A. Before treatment.
B. After treatment.

Case 2
A. Before treatment.
B. After treatment.

A Model Case Summary

A patient by name Ramesh aged 38 years, businessman in Bengaluru, reported to the Department of Periodontics with a chief complaint of bleeding gums from the past 3 months. No specific family or medical history was elicited. Past dental history revealed extraction of lower third molar due to dental caries and it was uneventful.

No relevant findings were observed on extraoral examination. Intraoral examination revealed generalized soft and edematous, gingiva with loss of stippling and bleeding on probing. Periodontal examination revealed average pocket depth of 5 mm, grade II furcation involvement with respect to mandibular first molar and grade I mobility with respect to 31, 32, 41, 42.

Based on above findings patient was diagnosed with chronic generalized periodontitis. Prognosis was established as fair. The treatment included phase I therapy re-evaluated for surgical phase.

Case 1A: Before treatment

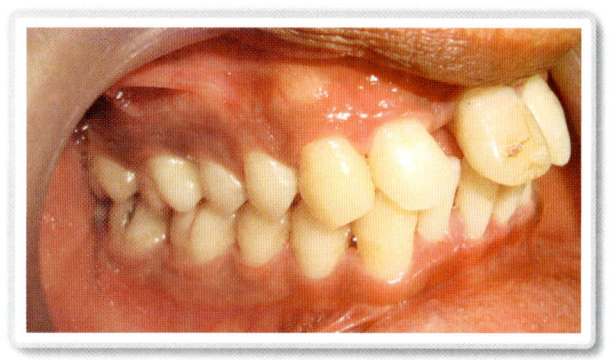

Case 1B: After treatment

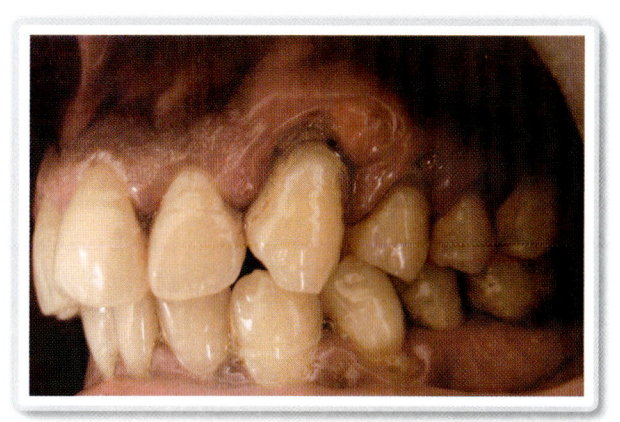

Case 2A: Before treatment

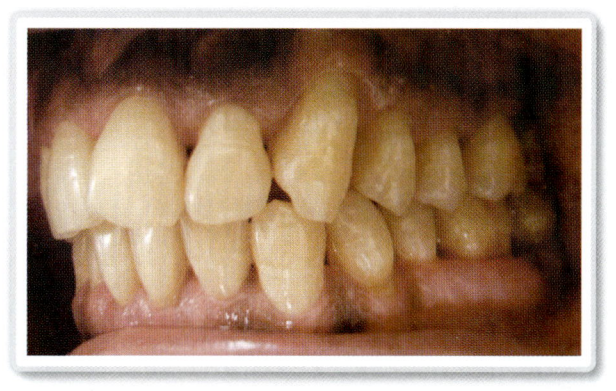

Case 2B: After treatment

CHAPTER 3

SECTION 2: Instrumentation

Periodontal Instruments and Instrumentation

PARTS OF PERIODONTAL INSTRUMENTS (Fig. 3.1)

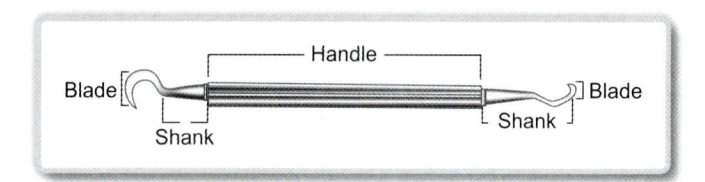

Fig. 3.1: Parts of an instrument

1. Blade: To perform specific tasks.
2. Handle: For grasping.
3. Shank: To gain sufficient access.

Types of Handle

- Hollow and solid
- Small and large
- Smooth, ribbed and knurled
- Diameter sizes available are 3/8, 5/16, 1/4 and 3/16 inches.

Types of Shank

- Rigid and flexible
- Straight and angled
- Short and long.

Types of Working Ends

Working end consists of face, back, lateral surface, cutting edge, heel, tip and toe.

Working Ends

1. Single ended has one working end.
2. Double ended has two working ends. It can be:
   a. Paired: Both ends are mirror images of each other.
   b. Complementary.

CLASSIFICATION OF PERIODONTAL INSTRUMENTS

1. Diagnostic instruments.
2. Scaling, root planing and curettage instruments:
   a. For supragingival scaling, sickle scalers, cumine universal scaler, posterior jacquette scaler, Morse scaler, surface scaler, cingulum scaler.
   b. For subgingival scaling:
      - Hoe scaler, chisel and file scalers
      - Curettes.
   c. Sonic and ultrasonic instruments.
3. Periodontal endoscope.
4. Cleansing and polishing instruments.
5. Surgical instruments.

DIAGNOSTIC INSTRUMENTS

Mouth Mirror

Design

Mouth mirror has three parts—handle, shank and working end (mirror head).

Three types of dental mirrors used are front surface (most commonly used, gives sharpest image), plane surface and magnifying surface.

Sizes

- 5/8 to 2 inch in diameter
- Handle sizes and shapes vary
- Angulation to shank and mirror vary; recommended is 45°.

Uses

Indirect vision, direct vision, retraction, illumination, transillumination.

Periodontal Probe

Design

Working end: It is blunt, straight and generally round and tapered with graduated millimeter markings.

Shank

- Junction between shank and working end is 90°
- Remaining shank can be straight or offset.

Types (Figs 3.2A to E and 3.3)

- Calibrated periodontal probe—color coded/non-color coded
- Nabers furcation probe.

Generations of Periodontal Probe (Refer Chapter 32)

Uses of Periodontal Probe

1. Used for recording pocket depth, attached gingiva, gingival recession.
2. For checking bleeding on probing.
3. Measurement of attached gingiva.
4. For determining shape, dimension and topography of gingival sulcus/periodontal pocket.
5. For location of calculus and furcation areas.
6. Checking dimensions of oral lesions.

Limitations of Conventional Probe

1. Periodontal probing fails to record the true pocket depth.
2. Factors which affect probing measurements are:
   a. Nature of soft tissues: In presence of gingival inflammation, there is overestimation of true pocket.

Fig. 3.3: Periodontal probes

   b. Probing force: Probes penetrate more deeply when high insertion forces used. Probing force varies from 3 to 130 g and accepted is 0.20–0.50 N.
   c. Size of the probe: Smaller diameter probe tips penetrate more deeply than larger diameter.
   d. Angulation of probe.
   e. Presence of calculus.
   f. Tooth morphology.
   g. Pocket configuration.
3. High interexaminer variability is seen.

Limitations of Automated Probes

1. Probing elements lack tactile sensitivity, mostly because of their independent movement, which forces the operator to predetermine an insertion point and angle.
2. Use of fixed force setting throughout the mouth, regardless of site or inflammation status, may generate inaccurate measurements or patients discomfort.
3. Underestimation of probing depth and clinical attachment levels by the automated probe.

Explorer

Design

Working end:
- Thin and tapered (tip)
- Single ended or double ended.

Shank: It can be straight, curved or angled.

Handle: It is light weighed to increase the tactile sensitivity.

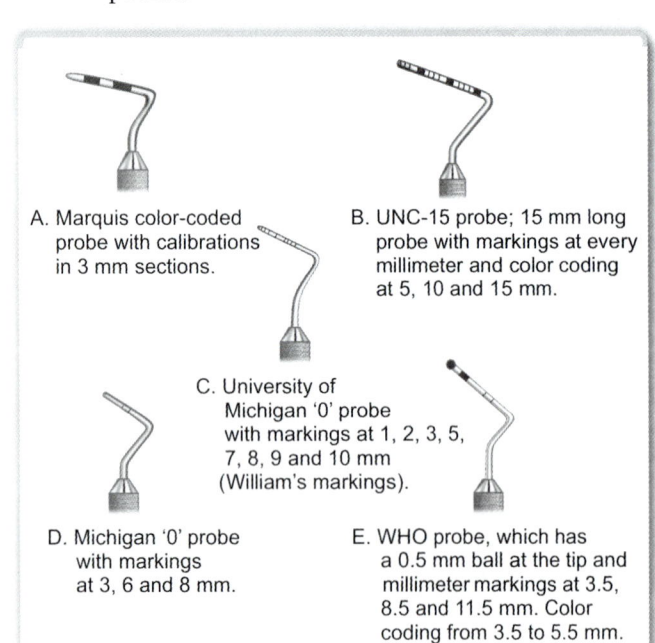

A. Marquis color-coded probe with calibrations in 3 mm sections.
B. UNC-15 probe; 15 mm long probe with markings at every millimeter and color coding at 5, 10 and 15 mm.
C. University of Michigan '0' probe with markings at 1, 2, 3, 5, 7, 8, 9 and 10 mm (William's markings).
D. Michigan '0' probe with markings at 3, 6 and 8 mm.
E. WHO probe, which has a 0.5 mm ball at the tip and millimeter markings at 3.5, 8.5 and 11.5 mm. Color coding from 3.5 to 5.5 mm.

Figs 3.2A to E: Different types of probes

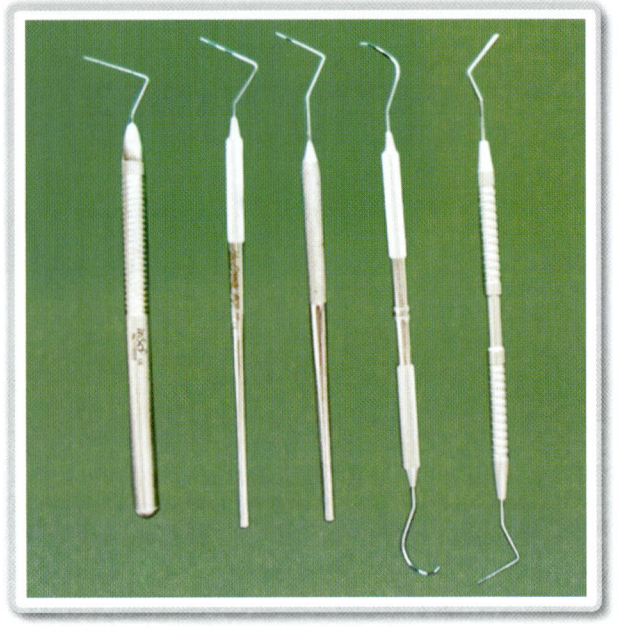

CHAPTER 3 Periodontal Instruments and Instrumentation

Types
- Shepherd's hook (No. 23)
- Pigtail/Cowhorn
- Orbans/No. 17
- 3A
- ODU 11/12.

Uses
1. To determine structure and surface characteristics of tooth surface.
2. For detection of caries, defective restoration, areas of decalcification.
3. For detection of amount and distribution of calculus.
4. Subgingivally for determining success of scaling and root planing, finishing of restorations and assessing root surface for cementum irregularities and diseases.

SCALING AND ROOT PLANING INSTRUMENTS

Scaling Instruments (Refer Fig. 3.9)

Supragingival Scalers
- Sickle scaler
- Morse scaler
- Surface scaler
- Cumine scaler.

Subgingival Scalers
- Hoe scaler
- Chisel scaler
- Periodontal file
- Islet scaler.

SUPRAGINGIVAL SCALERS

Sickle Scaler

Design (Figs 3.4 and 3.5)
1. It is triangular in cross-section, with a flat face.
2. The lateral surfaces meet the face to form two cutting edges and a pointed tip.
3. Face is perpendicular to the lower shank, so that cutting edges are in level with one another.
4. Shank:
   a. Anterior sickles: Simple design, straight shank.
   b. Posterior sickles: Complex design, angled shank.

Functions
1. Removal of medium- to large-sized supragingival calculus deposits.
2. Provides good access to the:
   a. Proximal surfaces on anterior crowns.
   b. Enamel surfaces apical to contact areas of posterior teeth. For example, anterior sickle scaler: OD-1, Jacquette-30 Jacquette-33, Towner-015, Goldman H6 and H7, Posterior sickle scalers: Jacquette 34/35, Jacquette 14/15, Jacquette 31/32, Ball 2/3.

Morse Scaler

Design

Small miniature blade.

Uses

Mandibular anterior area—narrow interproximal space. Sickle scalers vary in blade sizes and shank types, e.g. U15/30 has large blade and Jacquette scalers have

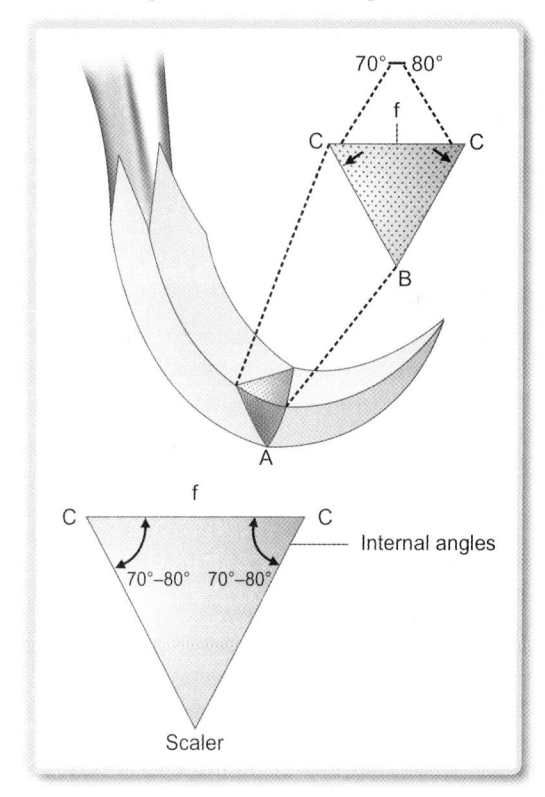

Fig. 3.4: Design of curved scaler (Sickle scaler)

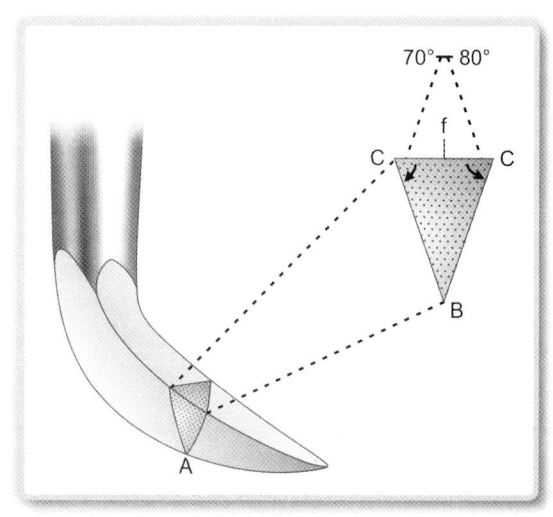

Fig. 3.5: Design of straight scaler (Jacquette scaler)

medium-sized blade. Morse scalers with small-sized blade (0, 00) are miniature instruments. Instruments with straight shank are used in anterior and premolars, and instruments with contra-angle are used on posterior teeth.

Surface Scaler

Use

Surface scaler is used for the removal of surface stains.

Cumine Scaler

Use

Cumine scaler is used for the removal of heavy, tenacious calculus.

The sharp-pointed end can be used for the removal of granulation tissue during periodontal flap surgeries.

SUBGINGIVAL SCALERS

Hoe Scaler

Design (Figs 3.6A to C)

1. Single blade at 99°–100° angle to terminal shank.
2. Single straight cutting edge beveled at 45° to the end of blade and forms at the junction of blade and toe.
3. Hoe has rounded back.
4. Single or double-ended instrument.

Types

McCall's Hoe scalers No. 3, 4, 5, 6, 7 and 8 are set of six hoe scalers.

Use

Heavy calculus removal—generally used in anterior sextant.

Chisel Scaler

Design (Figs 3.7A and B)

1. Single straight cutting edge.
2. Blade is continuous with the shank of the instrument and meets the 45° beveled toe to form cutting edge.
3. Blade has slight curvature to facilitate adaptation to proximal tooth surfaces.

Uses

1. Supragingival calculus removal in areas where interdental papilla is no longer present.
2. Used with push stroke.

Periodontal File

Design (Figs 3.8A and B)

1. Series of blades on base.
2. Base is rounded, oblong or rectangular.
3. Back is rounded to allow subgingival insertion.

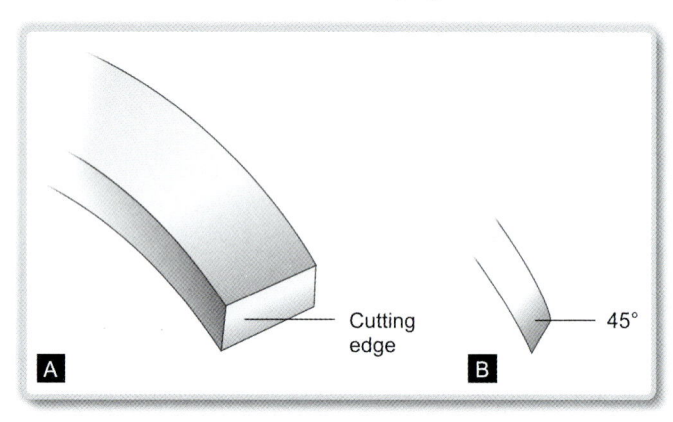

Figs 3.7A and B: Working end of chisel

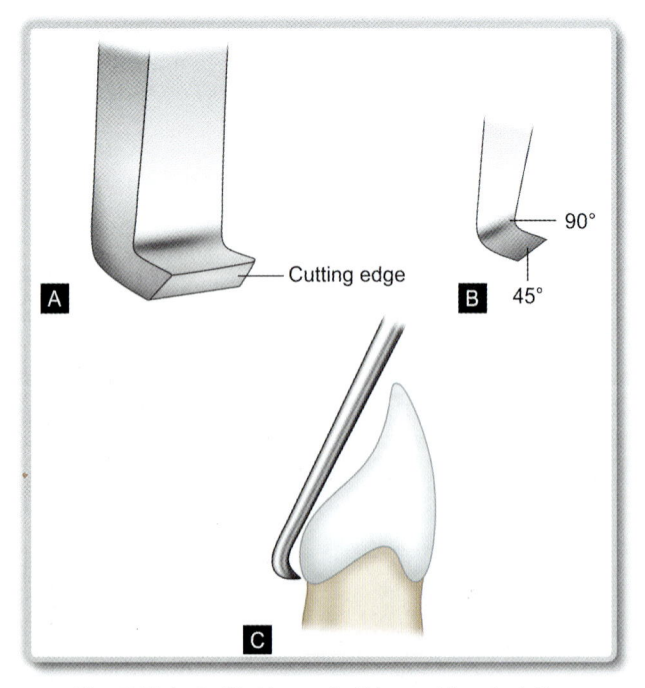

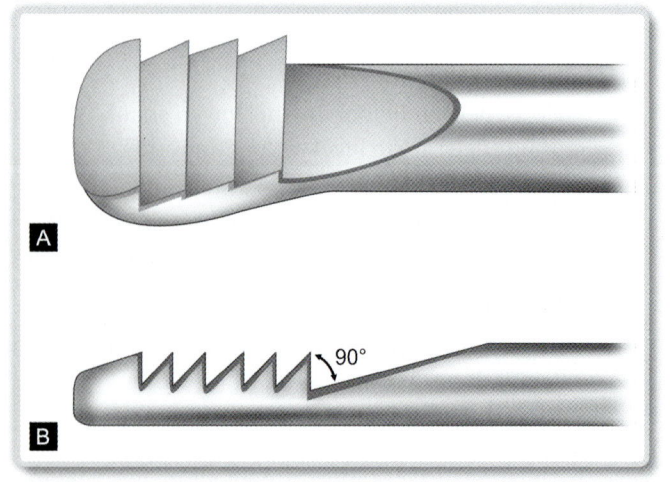

Figs 3.6A to C: Working end of Hoe and its adaptation to tooth surface

Figs 3.8A and B: Working end of file

4. Cutting edges are series of miniature hoes, which are set at approximately 90°–105° angle to base, which is approximately 55° angle between each blade.
5. Shank: It is heavy and rigid and can be straight or angled.
6. It can be single or double ended.

Uses

1. To smoothen cementoenamel junction/overhanging amalgam restoration.
2. *Technique:* Two point contact—for stability and leverage.
3. Used with pull stroke with moderate lateral pressure to crush calculus.

Islet Scaler

Use

Islet scaler is used for the removal of granulation tissue and necrotic cementum.

SUBGINGIVAL SCALING AND ROOT PLANING INSTRUMENTS

Curette is the instrument of choice for removing deep subgingival calculus; root planing, altered cementum and removing the soft tissue lining the periodontal pocket (Fig. 3.9).

These include:
- Universal curettes
- Area-specific curettes.
  In Gracey curettes (Fig. 3.10):
- 1-2 and 3-4: Anterior teeth
- 5-6: Anterior teeth and premolars
- 7-8 and 9-10: Posterior teeth facial and lingual
- 11-12: Posterior teeth (mesial)
- 13-14: Posterior teeth (distal).

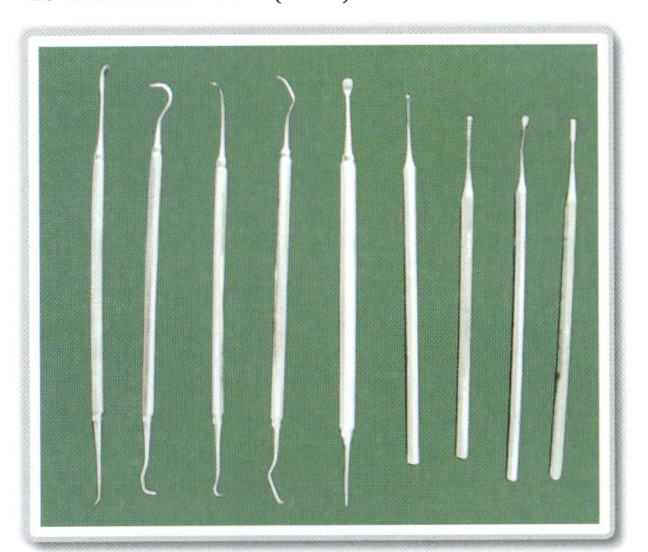

Fig. 3.9: Set of scaling instruments

ADVANCES IN ROOT PLANING INSTRUMENTS

1. *Gracey No. 15-16:* It is a modification of standard 11-12 and has an 11-12 blade with a 13-14 shank. It is useful for mesial surfaces of posterior teeth.
2. *Gracey No. 17-18:* It is a modification of standard 13-14. It is a 13-14 Gracey curette with a terminal shank elongated by 3 mm and a more accentuated angulation of shank.
3. *Extended shank curettes (after five curettes):* Here shank is elongated by 3 mm and is used for deeper periodontal pockets of 5 mm or more.
4. *Mini-bladed curettes (mini five curettes):* They are modifications of after five curettes with their blade reduced by half. It is used in furcation area, developmental grooves, tight pockets, deep narrow pockets.
5. *Gracey curettes:* Here, the blade length is half of the conventional Gracey curette and blade curves upwards.
6. *Langer and mini-Langer curettes:* It is a combination of universal and Gracey curettes available in 5-6, 11-12 and 13-14. It has similar shank design to a Gracey curette, but blade angle is 90 degrees.

Characteristics of Curette (Fig. 3.11)

	Universal	Area-specific
Cross-section	Semicircular	Semicircular
Back	Rounded	Rounded
Cutting edges	Two cutting edges	One cutting edge
Toe	Rounded	Rounded
Face	Perpendicular to the lower shank	Tilted at a 60°–70° to the lower shank

Contd...

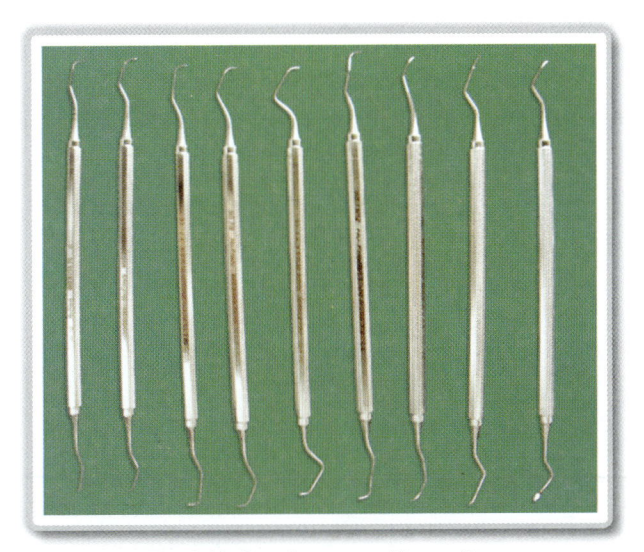

Fig. 3.10: Set of area-specific curettes

Contd...

	Universal	Area-specific
Application	Used to instrument all tooth surfaces in the dentition	Limited to use on a specific area of specific tooth surface
Function	Removal of light- to medium-sized calculus deposits	Removal of light calculus deposits
Examples	Columbia 2R/2L, Columbia 13/14, Rule 3/4, Barnhart 1/2 Barnhart 5/6 Langer 1/2 Langer 3/4 Langer 5/6 Langer 17/18	Gracey series Kramer-Nevins series Turgeon series After five Mini five Vision curette series

Differences Between Universal and Gracey Curettes (Figs 3.12 and 3.14)

	Gracey curette	Universal curette
Area of use	Set of many curettes designed for specific areas and surfaces	One curette designed for all areas and surfaces
Cutting edge use	One cutting edge used; work with outer edge only	Both cutting edges used work with either outer or inner edge
Curvature	Curved in two planes; blade curves up and to the side	Curved in one plane; blade curves up, not to side
Blade angle	Offset blade; face of blade beveled at 60° to shank	Not offset; face of blade beveled at 90° to shank

Differences Between Scaler and Curette (Figs 3.12 and 3.13)

	Scaler	Universal curette
Cross-section	Triangular in cross-section	Semicircular cross-section
Working end	Pointed back and tip Two cutting edges per working end	Rounded back and toe Two cutting edges per working end
Face	Face is perpendicular to lower shank	Face is at 90° angle to the lower shank Two parallel cutting edges meet in a rounded toe
Application	Anterior teeth only one single ended instrument is needed Post-teeth—one double ended instrument is needed	Universal use
Primary function	Removal of medium- to large-sized supragingival calculus	Debridement of crown and root surfaces Removal of small- to medium-sized calculus deposits

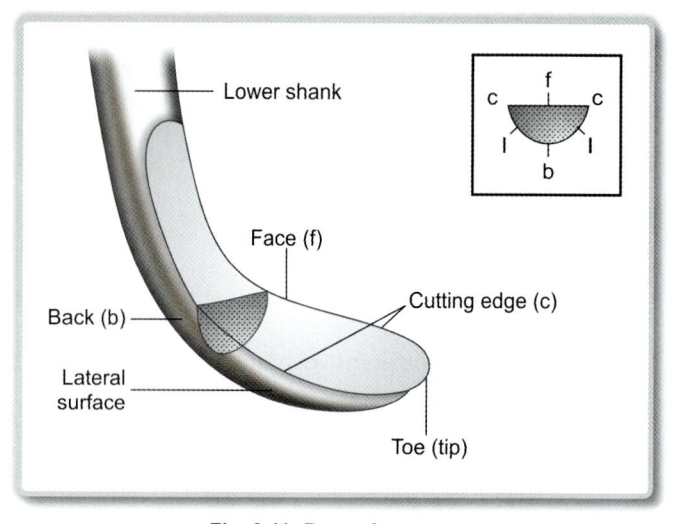

Fig. 3.11: Parts of a curette

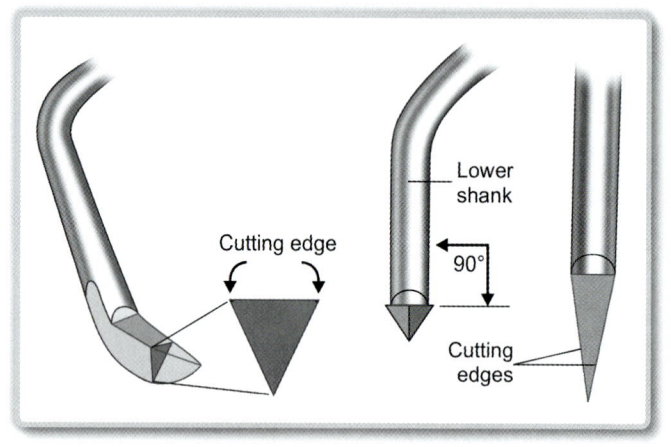

Fig. 3.12: Working end of scaler

PRINCIPLES OF PERIODONTAL INSTRUMENTATION

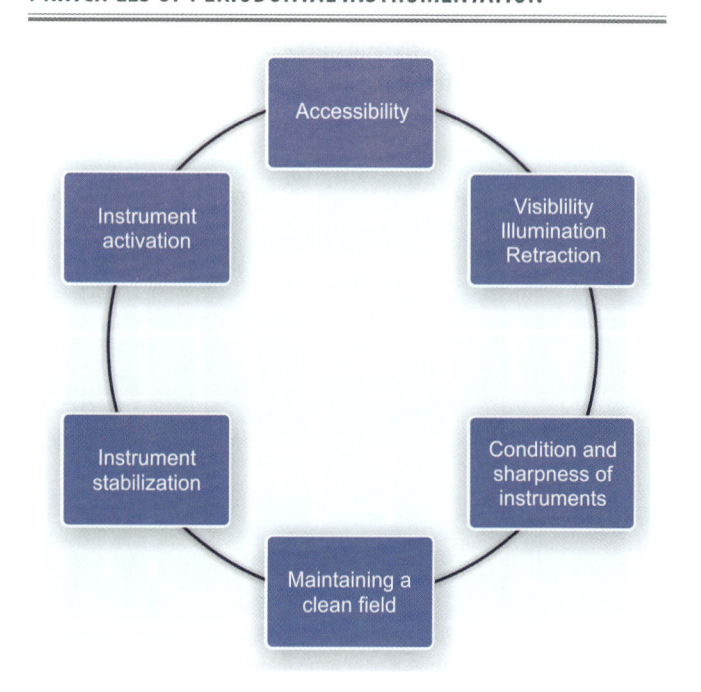

- Accessibility
- Visiblility Illumination Retraction
- Condition and sharpness of instruments
- Maintaining a clean field
- Instrument stabilization
- Instrument activation

Accessibility

Positioning of the Patient and Operator (Figs 3.15 to 3.21)

It facilitates thoroughness of instrumentation. The position of the patient and operator should provide maximal accessibility to the area of operation:

1. Forearms should be parallel to the floor.
2. Weight evenly balanced.
3. Thighs parallel to the floor.
4. Hip angle of 90 degree.
5. Seat height positioned low enough so that you are able to rest the heels of your feet on the floor.

Permissible (Fig. 3.16)

1. Head should be tilted between 0° and 15°.
2. The line from eyes to the treatment area should be as near to vertical as possible.

Avoid

1. Head should not be tipped too far forward.
2. Head should not be tilted to one side.

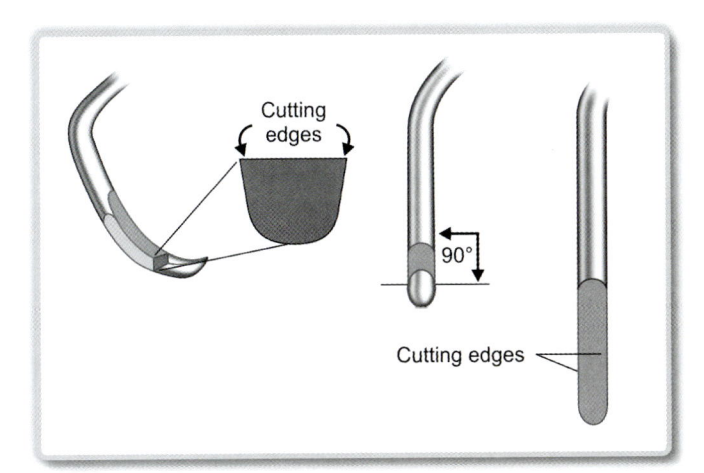

Fig. 3.13: Working end of universal curette

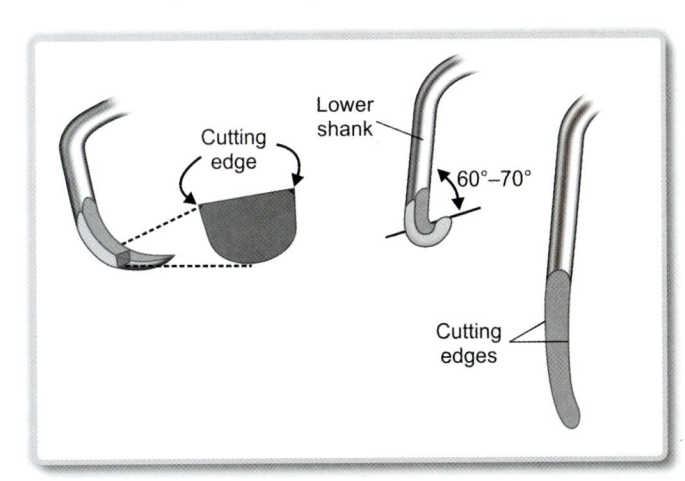

Fig. 3.14: Working end of area-specific curette

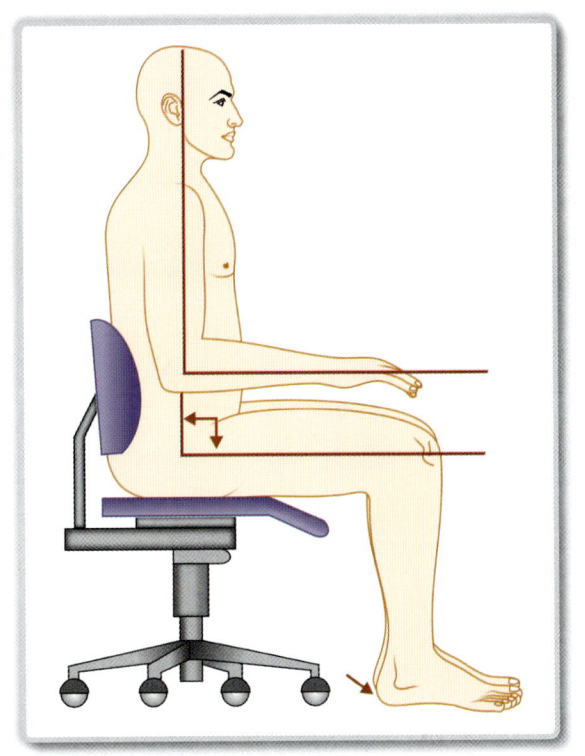

Fig. 3.15: Neutral seated position for the clinician

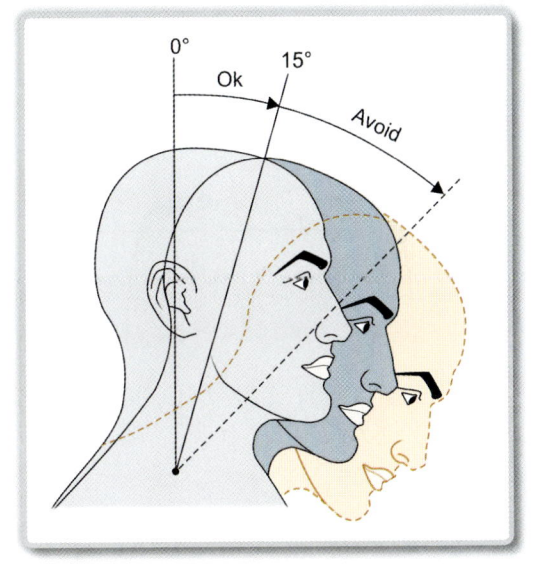

Fig. 3.16: Neutral neck position

Permissible (Fig. 3.17)

1. Leaning forward slightly from the waist or hips.
2. Trunk flexion of 0°–20°.

Avoid

Overflexion of the spine (curved back).

Permissible (Fig. 3.18)

1. Shoulders should be in horizontal line.
2. Weight should be evenly balanced when seated.

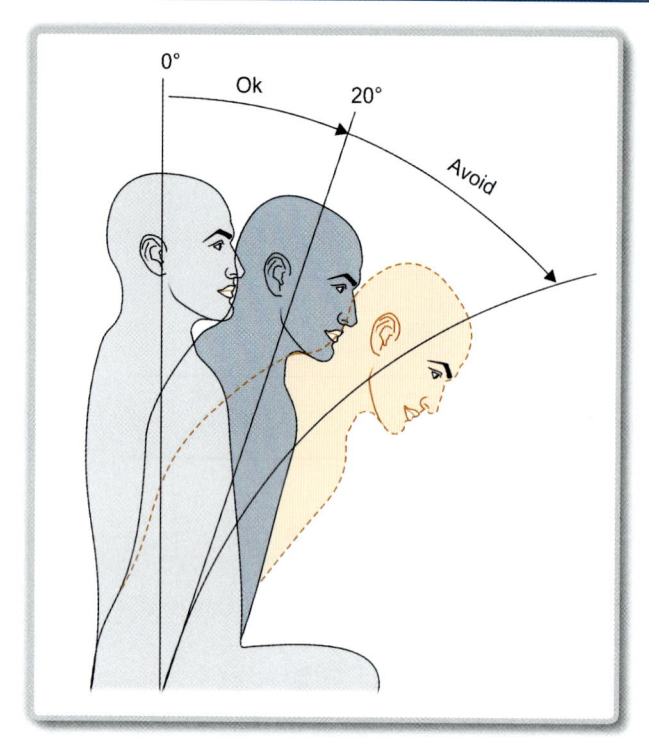

Fig. 3.17: Neutral back position

2. Elbows should be at waist level and held slightly away from the body.

Avoid

1. Elbows more than 20° away from the body.
2. Elbows held above the waist level.

Permissible (Fig. 3.20)

1. Forearms should be parallel to the floor.

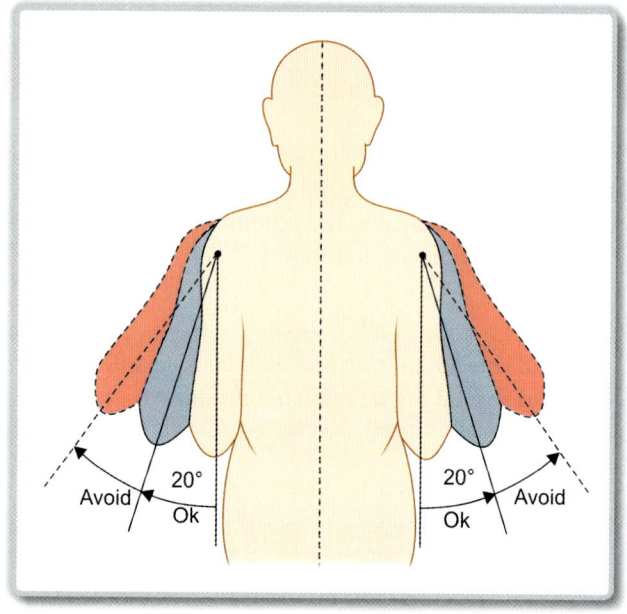

Fig. 3.19: Neutral upper arm position

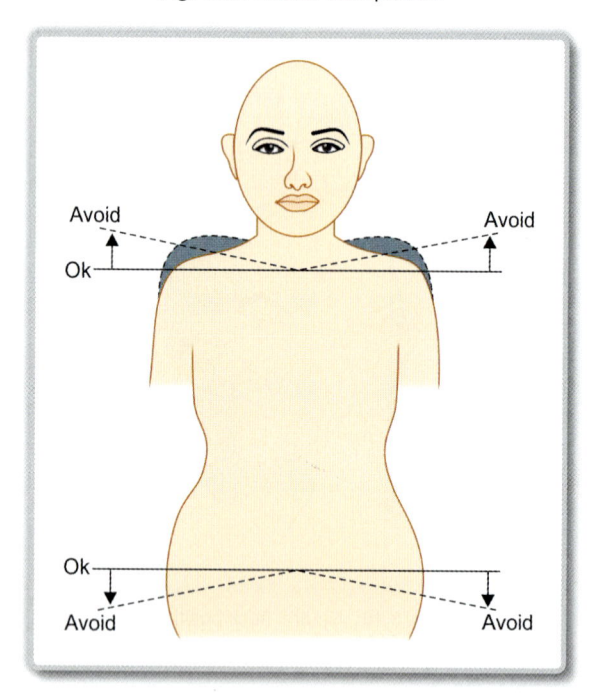

Fig. 3.18: Neutral shoulder position

Avoid

1. Shoulders lifted up toward the ears.
2. Shoulders hunched forward.
3. Sitting with weight on one hip.

Permissible (Fig. 3.19)

1. Upper arms should hang parallel to the long axis of torso.

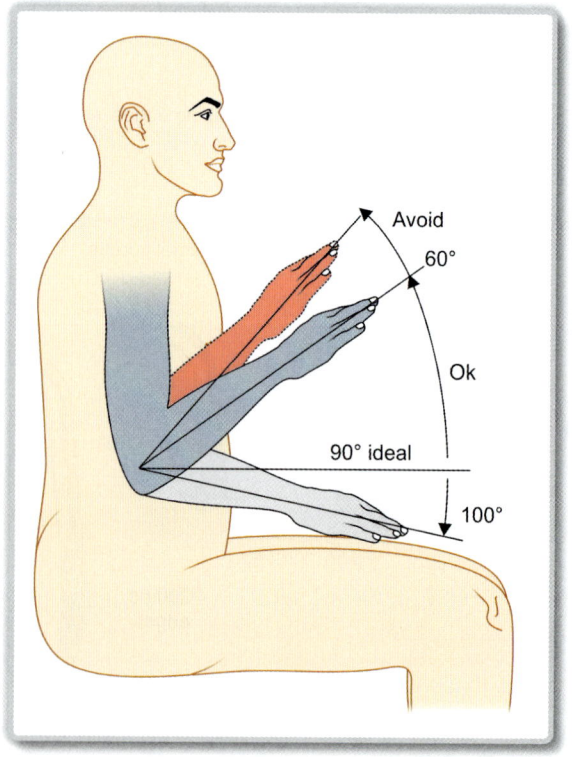

Fig. 3.20: Neutral forearm position

2. Forearms should be raised or lowered, if necessary, by pivoting at the elbow joint.

Avoid

Angle between forearm and upper arm lesser than 60°.

Permissible (Fig. 3.21A)

1. Little finger side of the palm should be slightly lower than thumb side of the palm.
2. Wrist should be aligned with the forearm.

Avoid

1. Thumb side of the palm should not be rotated down so that palm is parallel to the floor.
2. Hand or wrist should not be bent up or down.

RECOMMENDED POSITION (Fig. 3.21B)

Body

The patient's heels should be slightly higher than the tip of the nose. This position maintains a good blood flow to the head. An apprehensive patient is more likely to faint if positioned with the head higher than the heel. The chair back should be nearly parallel to the floor for the maxillary treatment areas. The chair back may be raised slightly for mandibular treatment areas (Table 3.1).

TABLE 3.1: Positioning summary for a right-handed clinician (Fig. 3.22)

Treatment area	Clock position	Patient head position
Mandibular arch—Anterior surfaces toward	8:00–9:00	Slightly toward, **chin-down**
Maxillary arch—Anterior surfaces toward	8:00–9:00	Slightly toward, **chin-up**
Mandibular arch—Anterior surfaces away	12:00	Slightly toward, **chin-down**
Maxillary arch—Anterior surfaces away	12:00	Slightly toward, **chin-up**
Mandibular arch—Posterior aspects facing toward	9:00	Slightly away, **chin-down**
Maxillary arch—Posterior aspects facing toward	9:00	Slightly away, **chin-up**
Mandibular arch—Posterior aspects facing toward	10:00–11:00	Toward, **chin-down**
Maxillary arch—Posterior aspects facing toward	10:00–11:00	Toward, **chin-up**

Head

The top of the patient's head should be even with upper edge of the head rest. If necessary, ask the patient to slide up in the chair to assume this position.

Head Rest

If the head rest is adjustable raise or lower it so that the patient's neck and head are aligned with the torso.

BASIC POSITIONING OF THE PATIENT'S HEAD

Recommended Position

Position on the Head Rest

To be able to see and reach the patient's mouth comfortably, the top of the patient's head must be even with the end of the head rest.

Mandibular Areas

Ask the patient to open the mouth and tilt the head downward. The term for this patient head position is the ***chin-down position.***

Maxillary Areas

Ask the patient to open the mouth and position the head in a neutral position. The term for the patient head position is the chin-up position.

VISIBILITY, ILLUMINATION AND RETRACTION (Figs 3.23 and 3.24)

Whenever possible, direct vision with direct illumination from the dental light is most desirable. If this is not possible, indirect vision may be obtained using mouth mirror to

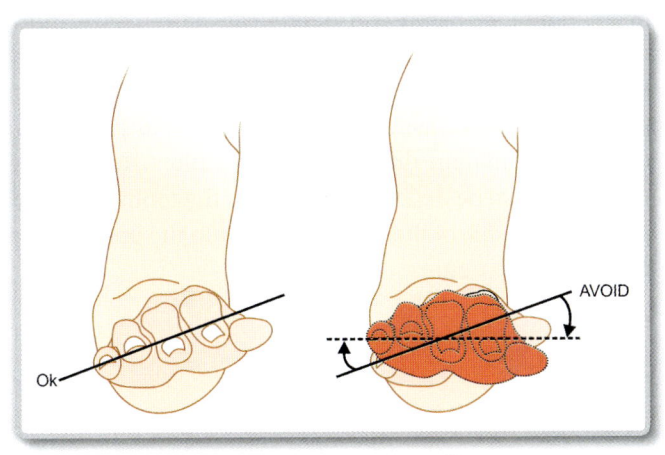

Fig. 3.21A: Neutral hand position

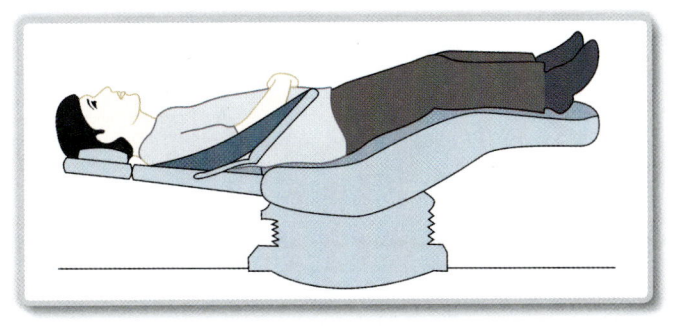

Fig. 3.21B: The supine patient position

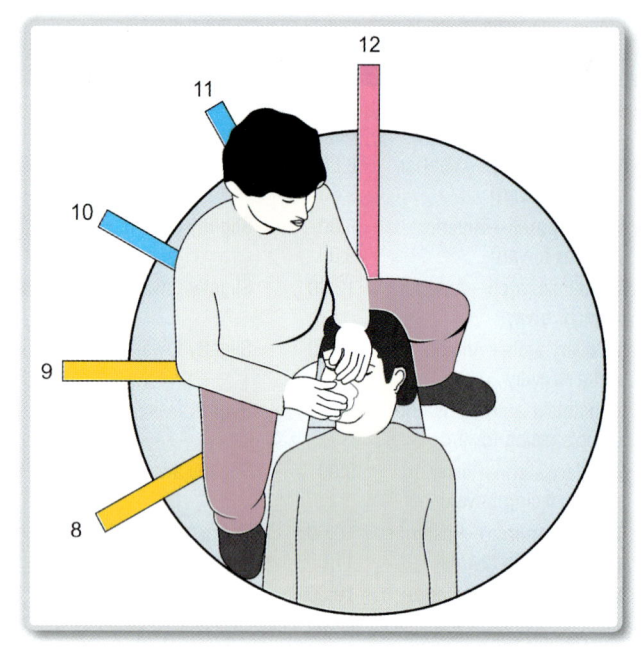

Fig. 3.22: Clock positions for right-handed clinician

reflect light where it is needed. Indirect vision and indirect illumination are often used simultaneously.

TRANSILLUMINATION

When transilluminating a tooth, a mouth mirror is used to reflect light through the tooth surface. The transilluminated tooth will appear to glow.

Dental light: Position dental light directly above the patient's head. Light should be as far as possible, while still remaining within easy reach. In this position, the light beam will shine directly down into the patient's mouth (Fig. 3.25).

Dental light: Position the dental light above the patient's chest. Tilt the light, so that the light beam shines into the patient's mouth at an angle. Position the light as far away from the patient's face as possible, while still keeping it within easy reach (Fig. 3.26).

Retraction

This can be done by:
1. Use of the mirror to deflect the cheek while fingers of the non-operating hand retract the lips and protect the angle of the mouth from irritation by the mirror handle.
2. Use of the mirror alone to retract lips and cheek.
3. Use of fingers of the non-operating hand to retract the lips.
4. Use of the mirror to retract the tongue.
5. Combination of the preceding methods.

CONDITION OF INSTRUMENTS (SHARPNESS)

Advantages of Instrument Sharpness
- Easier calculus removal
- Improved stroke control
- Reduced number of strokes
- Increased patient comfort
- Reduced clinician fatigue.

MAINTAINING A CLEAN FIELD

Maintaining a clean field can be achieved by saliva ejector or an aspirator. Blood and debris can be removed from the operative field with suction and by blotting with gauze squares. Compressed air and gauze squares can be used to facilitate visual inspection of tooth surfaces just below the gingival margin during instrumentation. Retractable tissue can also be deflected away from the tooth by gently packing the edge of the gauze square into the pocket with the back of a curette.

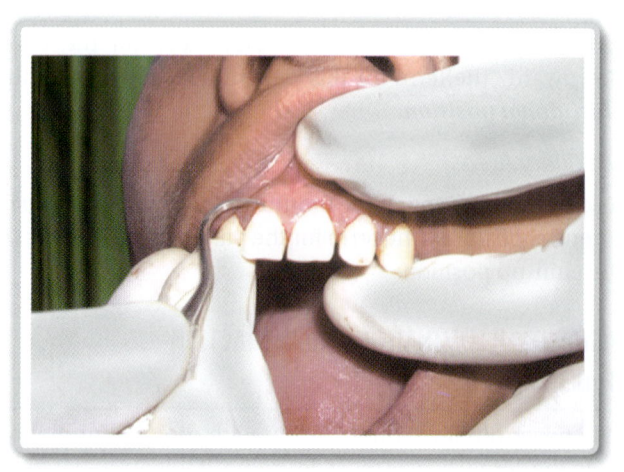

Fig. 3.23: Direct visibility

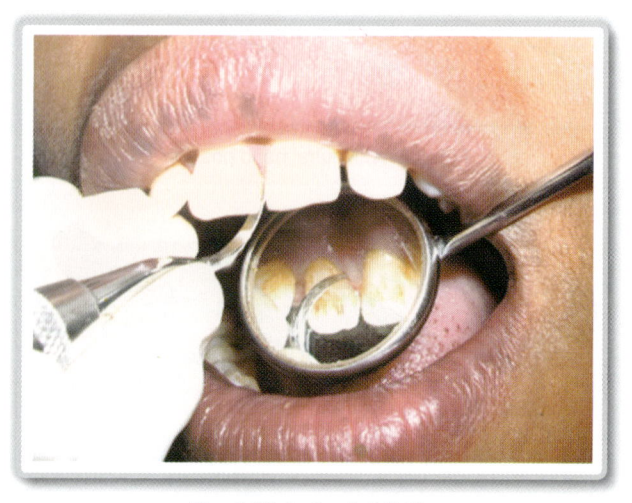

Fig. 3.24: Indirect visibility

CHAPTER 3 Periodontal Instruments and Instrumentation

Instrument Grasps (Figs 3.27 to 3.29)

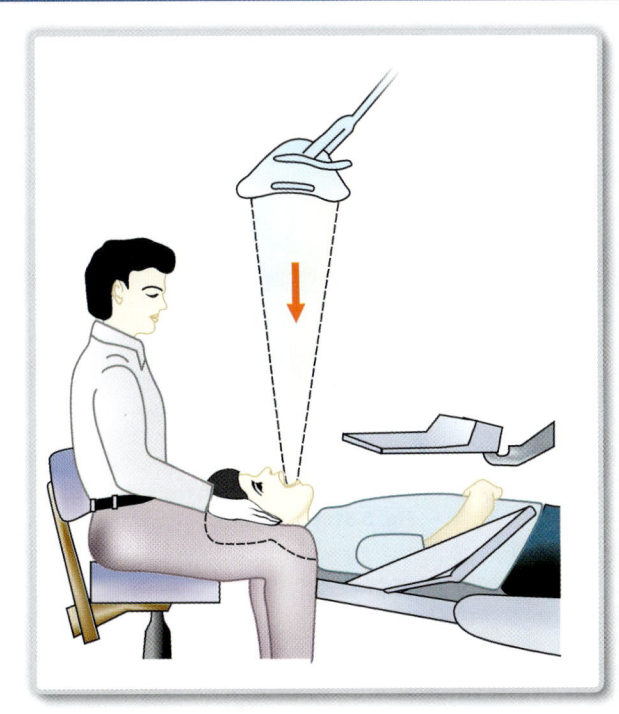

Fig. 3.25: Light position for mandibular teeth

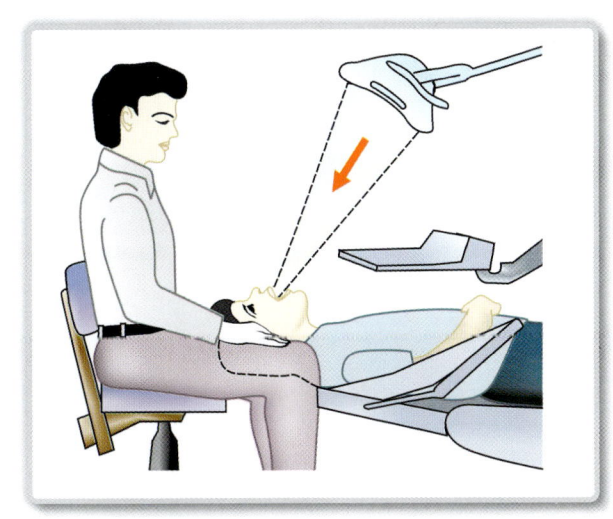

Fig. 3.26: Light position for maxillary teeth

INSTRUMENT STABILIZATION

Two factors that provide stability are instrument grasp and finger rest (Table 3.2).

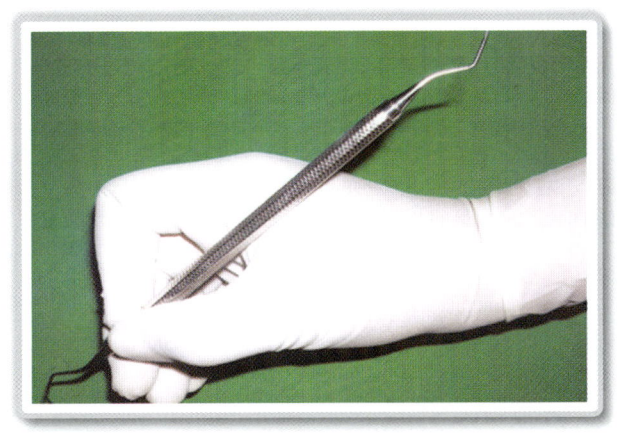

Fig. 3.27: Pen grasp

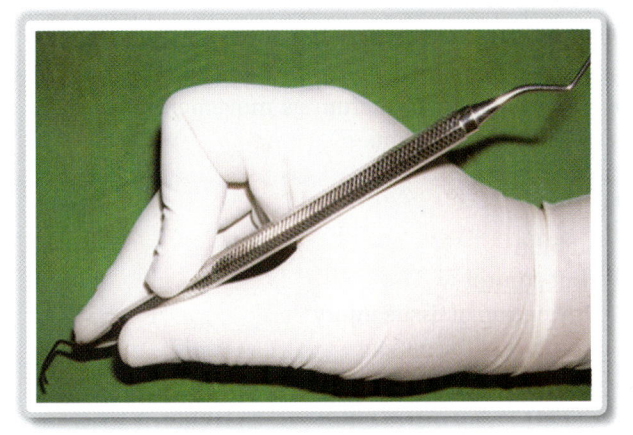

Fig. 3.28: Modified pen grasp

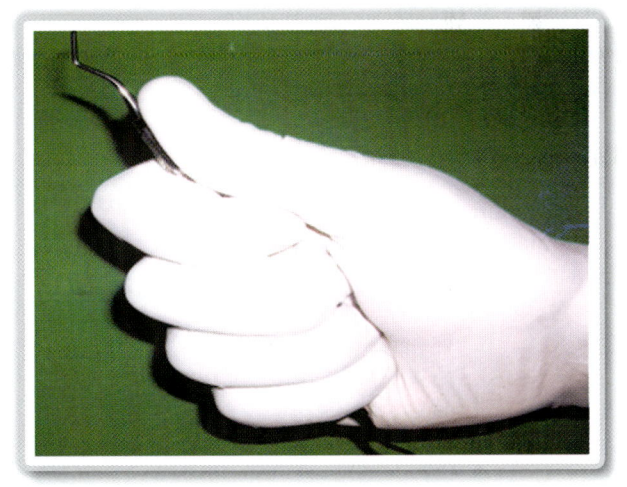

Fig. 3.29: Palm and thumb grasp

TABLE 3.2:	Correct finger placement
Digit	Recommended position and function
Thumb and index	The finger pads rest opposite to each other at or near the junction of the handle and the shank. They do not overlap and a tiny space exists between them. The instrument is held in a relaxed manner. The index finger and thumb curve outward from the handle in a C-shape. The main function of these digits is to hold the instrument.
Middle	One side of the finger pad rests lightly on the instrument shank. The other side of the finger pad rests against the ring finger. It helps to guide the working end and also feel the vibration.
Ring	Fingertip balances firmly on the tooth to support the weight of the hand and instrument. The finger is held straight and upright to act as a strong support beam for the hand.
Little	It should be held in a relaxed manner with no function.

Finger Rest

Finger rest serves to stabilize the hand and the instrument by providing a firm fulcrum as movements are made to activate the instrument.

Objectives

- Stability
- Unit control
- Prevention of tissue injury
- Comfort of the patient
- Control of length of stroke.

Intraoral and Extraoral Finger Rests (Figs 3.30 to 3.35)

The intraoral finger rest is essentially a hand coordinated effort to provide stabilization.

INSTRUMENT ACTIVATION

- Adaptation
- Angulation

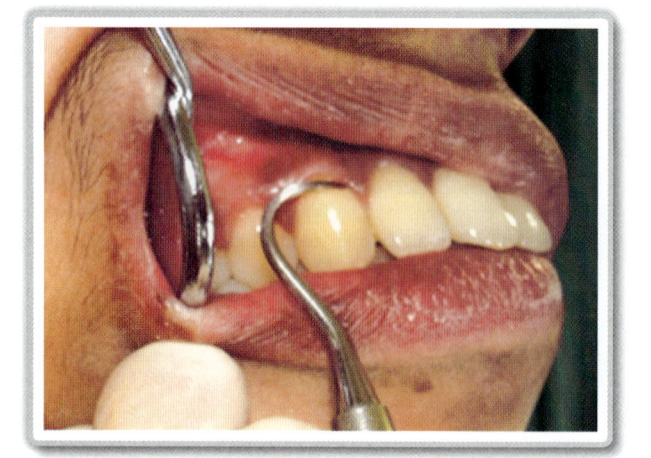

Fig. 3.30: Palm up

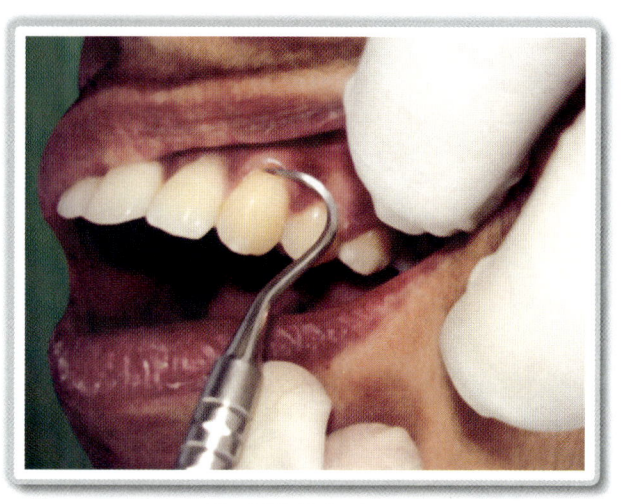

Fig. 3.31: Palm down

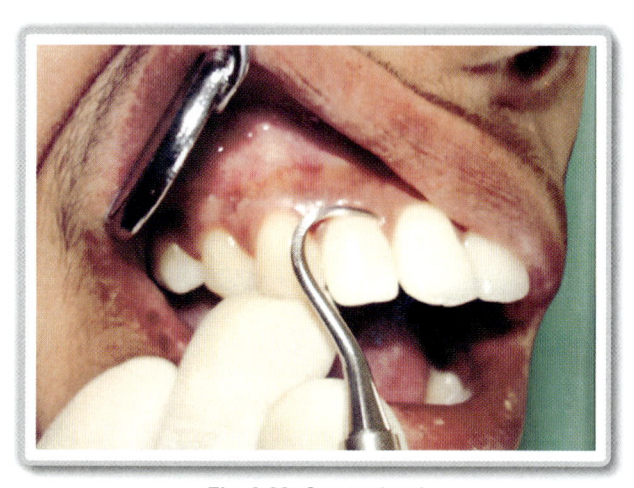

Fig. 3.32: Conventional

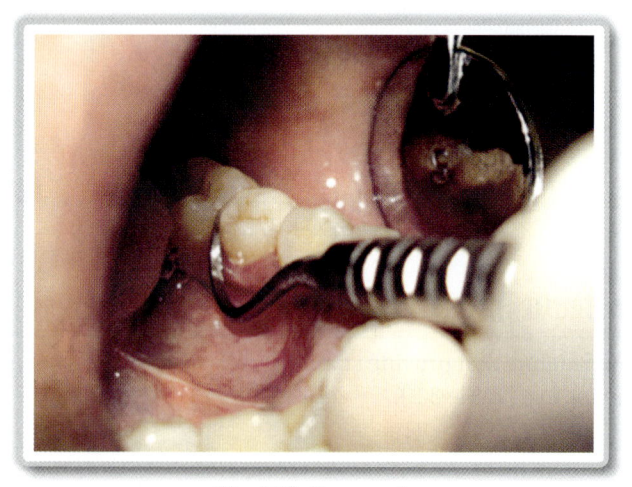

Fig. 3.33: Cross arch

- Lateral pressure
- Strokes.

Adaptation

Adaptation refers to the manner in which the working end of a periodontal instrument is placed against the tooth

CHAPTER 3 Periodontal Instruments and Instrumentation

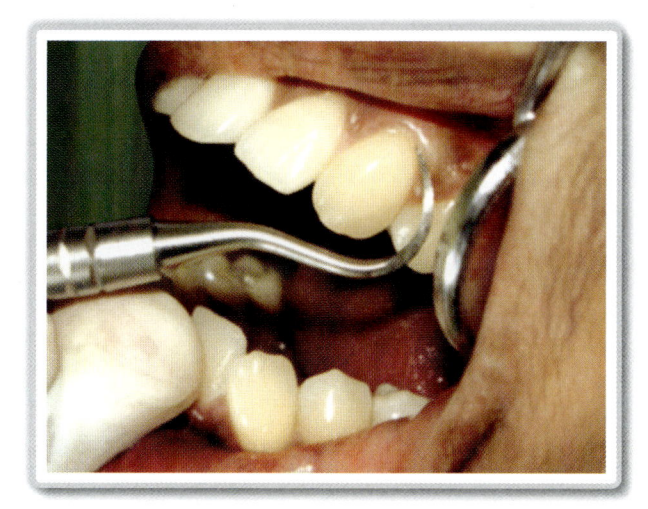

Fig. 3.34: Opposite arch

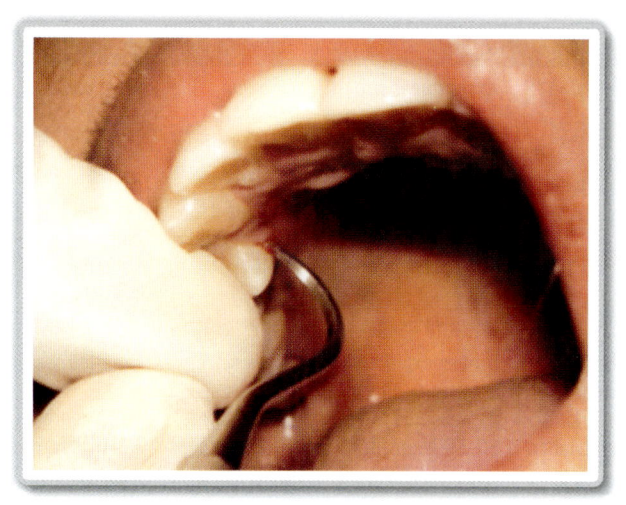

Fig. 3.35: Finger on finger

surface. The objective of adaptation is to make the working end of the instrument to conform with the contour of the tooth.

Angulation (Fig. 3.36)

Angulation refers to the angle between the face of a bladed instrument and the tooth surface.

LATERAL PRESSURE

Lateral pressure means the pressure of the instrument against the tooth surface during activation. It is described as light, moderate or heavy pressure.

Types

- Assessment stroke
- Scaling stroke or working stroke
- Root planing stroke
- Root debridement stroke.

Activation

Stroke

A stroke is an unbroken movement made by an instrument; it is the action of an instrument in the performance of the task for which it was designed (Table 3.3).

TYPES OF STROKE BY DIRECTION (Fig. 3.37)

- Diagonal or oblique stroke
- Vertical stroke
- Horizontal stroke.

To summarize, the principles of periodontal instrumentation, the ten commandments should be followed during supragingival hand scaling as given below:

1. Direct vision is desirable, but it is always better to visualize the area with indirect vision focusing on all the surfaces to identify the presence of calculus.

   Note: Identifying the calculus deposits is most essential for successful scaling procedure.

2. While adapting the instrument, the tip of the scaler should be placed away from the soft tissues.
3. The tip of the instrument should be mostly pointing downwards for the upper teeth and upwards for the lower teeth (Fig. 3.38).
4. Do not try and adapt the cutting edge of the instrument along the entire cervical portion, then the tip of the instrument will invariably contact the papilla and can cause the tissue damage.
5. The cervical portion should be divided into mesial and distal halves and the instrumentation should be done accordingly.
6. Interproximally, it is more challenging to perform scaling because, the calculus may be attached to the

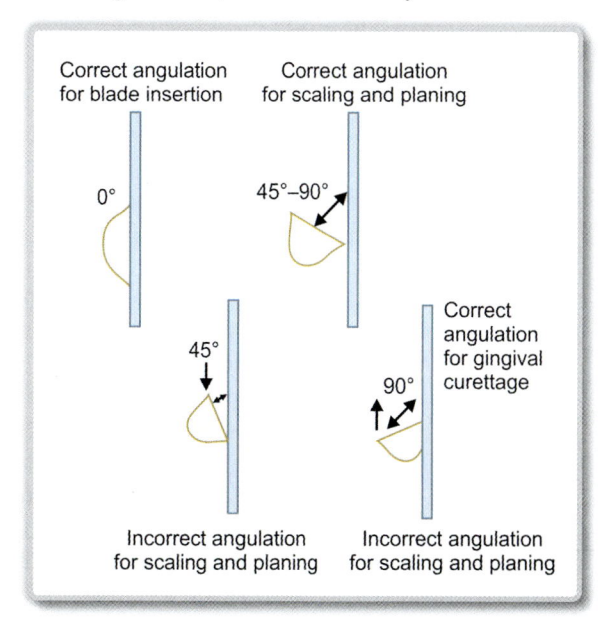

Fig. 3.36: Instrument angulation

TABLE 3.3:	Characteristics of strokes		
	Assessment stroke	*Calculus removal/ Scaling stroke*	*Root planing stroke*
Purpose	Assess tooth anatomy Level of attachment Detect calculus and other plaque retentive factors	Remove calculus deposits	Remove residual calculus, bacterial plaque and byproducts
Used with insertion Working angulation	Probes/explorers, curettes 0–40 degrees 50–70 degrees	Sickle scalers, curettes, files 0–40 degrees 70–80 degrees	Curettes 0–40 degrees 60–70 degrees
Lateral pressure	Contacts tooth surface, but no pressure applied	Moderate to firm scraping	Light to moderate
Character	Fluid stroke of moderate length	Powerful strokes short in length	Lighter strokes of moderate length
Direction	Vertical, oblique, horizontal	Vertical, oblique, horizontal	Vertical, oblique,
Number	Many, covering entire root surface	Limited, to area where needed	Many, covering entire root surface

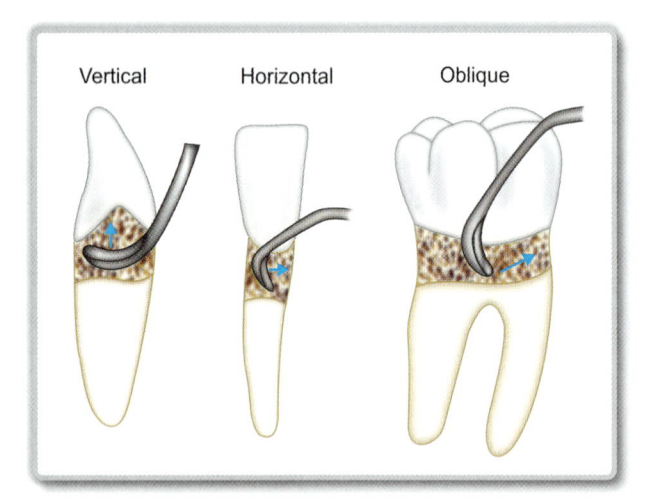

Fig. 3.37: Types of instrument strokes

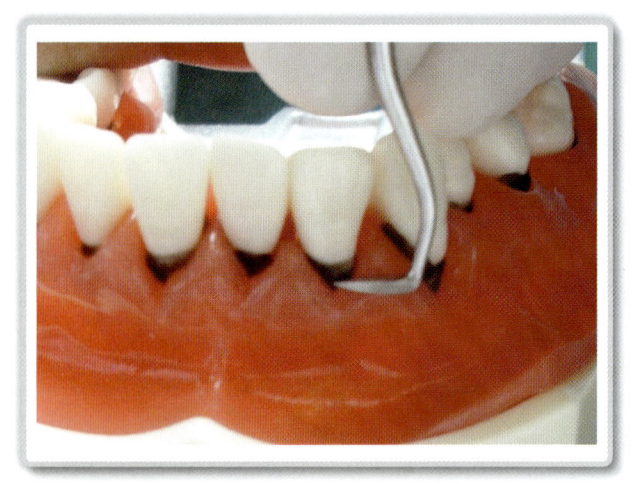

Fig. 3.38: Instrument adaptation on lower anteriors

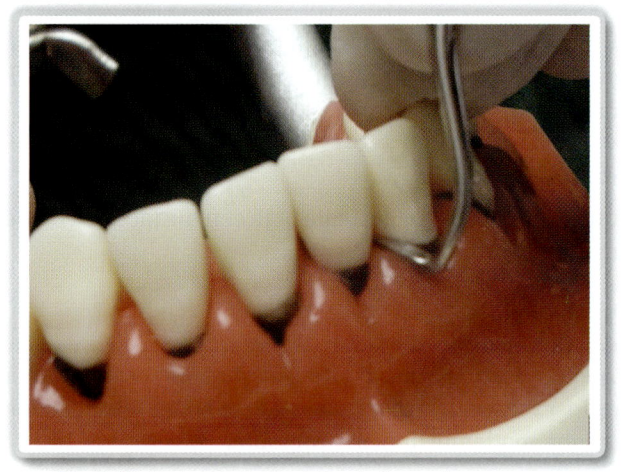

Fig. 3.39: Instrument adaptation in the embrasure area

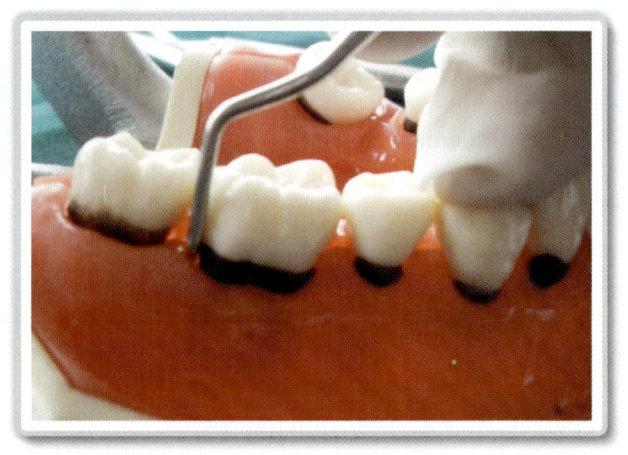

Fig. 3.40: Instrument adaptation in the posterior embrasure area

proximal surfaces of two adjacent teeth, as well as it may fill the entire embrasure area. Keep this in mind, while performing interdental scaling.

7. It is just not enough to remove the calculus from only the embrasure areas, the proximal surfaces also need to be scaled especially in the lower anterior teeth where the embrasures are narrow. In these situations, the best way to perform scaling is to detach the calculus from both the labial and lingual surfaces simultaneously (Figs 3.39 and 3.40).

8. Any type of finger rest can be utilized, but what is important is that, the finger rest should remain in place throughout the entire scaling stroke, i.e. do not displace the finger while instrument is being activated (no freehand scaling).

9. Instrument should be adapted to engage the base of calculus (below the undercut) get a firm grip and then perform the scaling stroke, this will avoid burnishing of the calculus.

10. Scaling is never complete, unless and until one systematically checks all the surfaces (mesial, distal, buccal, palatal/lingual) through direct and indirect vision for any remnants of calculus.

CHAPTER 4

SECTION 3: Viva Voce

Anatomy and Development of the Structures of Periodontium

Q1. Define periodontology.

Answer

The clinical science that deals with the periodontium in health and disease is called periodontology.

Q2. Define periodontics or periodontia.

Answer

The branch of dentistry concerned with prevention and treatment of periodontal disease.

Q3. What are the components of periodontium?

Answer

The periodontium is composed of the following tissues namely alveolar bone, root cementum, periodontal ligament (supporting tissues) and gingiva (investing tissues).

Q4. Enumerate the three zones of oral mucosa? Describe the parts of gingiva.

Answer

1. Masticatory mucosa: It includes the gingiva and covering of the hard palate.
2. Specialized mucosa: It covers the dorsum of the tongue.
3. Lining mucosa: Is the oral mucous membrane that lines the remainder of the oral cavity.

Q5. How is gingiva divided anatomically?

Answer

The gingiva is divided anatomically into free or marginal, attached and interdental gingiva.

Q6. What is free gingival groove?

Answer

The border or groove between marginal and attached gingiva is called a free gingival groove, a shallow depression on the faciogingival surface that roughly corresponds to the base of the gingival sulcus.

Q7. What is mucogingival junction?

Answer

The junction between the attached gingiva and alveolar mucosa is called mucogingival line or junction.

Q8. What is normal color of gingiva?

Answer

The normal gingiva is pink in color (salmon coral pink).

Q9. What is stippling?

Answer

The surface of the gingiva exhibits an orange peel-like appearance referred as stippling.

Q10. What is interdental gingiva? Where it is present?

Answer

The gingiva that completely fills the spaces between the teeth is known as interdental gingival. It is present in the posterior teeth, where the contact areas between the teeth are usually broad. The interdental gingiva consists of two papillae, facial and lingual which are connected by the col.

Q11. What is the significance of col?

Answer

The significance of col is that, it is made up of non-keratinized epithelium and hence represents the most frequent site for initiation of disease process.

Q12. How is Hertwig's epithelial root sheath formed? What is its function?

Answer

The outer and inner epithelia together form the epithelial root sheath of Hertwig, which is responsible for determining the shape of the root.

Q13. What is reduced enamel epithelium? What is its significance?

Answer

Once the crown formation is complete, the cells of the inner enamel epithelium lose their ability to form enamel and is called reduced enamel epithelium. They retain the ability to induce perimesenchymal cells to differentiate into odontoblasts and to proceed with the formation of predentin and dentin.

Q14. What is hyaline layer of Hopewell-Smith or intermediate cementum?

Answer

The epithelial cells of root sheath produce a layer on the dentin, which is 10 microns thick, has a hyaline appearance and contain granules and fibrils. This layer is called the hyaline layer of Hopewell-Smith or intermediate cementum.

Q15. What are enameloids or amelogenin?

Answer

The epithelial cells of the root sheath secrete enamel proteins and these are called enameloids or amelogenin.

Q16. What are Sharpey's fibers?

Answer

Sharpey's fibers are the terminal ends of principal fibers (of the periodontal ligament) that insert into the cementum and into the periosteum of the alveolar bone.

Q17. How is junctional epithelium formed?

Answer

Fusion of the oral epithelium along with the reduced enamel epithelium gives rise to the junctional epithelium.

CHAPTER 5

Biology of Periodontal Tissues

Q1. Define periodontium.

Answer

The tissues that invest and support the teeth including the gingiva, alveolar mucosa, cementum, periodontal ligament and alveolar bone.

Q2. What is dentoperiodontal unit?

Answer

The tooth and periodontium are together called the dentoperiodontal unit.

Q3. Define gingiva.

Answer

The gingiva is that part of the oral mucosa (masticatory mucosa) that covers the alveolar process of the jaws and surrounds the neck of the teeth.

Q4. Define marginal gingiva or free gingiva or unattached gingiva.

Answer

It is defined as the terminal edge or border of the gingiva surrounding the teeth in a collar-like fashion.

Q5. Define gingival sulcus.

Answer

It is defined as the space or shallow crevice between the tooth and free gingiva.

Q6. What is the normal probing depth of gingival sulcus clinically?

Answer

Probing depth of a clinically-normal gingival sulcus in humans is 2–3 mm.

Q7. Define attached gingiva.

Answer

It is defined as that part of the gingiva that is firm, resilient and tightly-bound to the underlying periosteum of the alveolar bone. It is continuous with the marginal gingiva and extends up to the alveolar mucosa.

Q8. Define the width of attached gingiva.

Answer

The width of attached gingiva is the distance between the mucogingival junction and the projection on the external surface of the bottom of the gingival sulcus or the periodontal pocket. It is greatest in the incisor region, i.e. 3.5–4.5 mm in maxilla and 3.3 mm in the mandible. It is least in the posterior segment 1.9 mm in maxilla and 1.8 mm in mandibular premolar region.

Q9. What are the cell layers present in the oral epithelium?

Answer

The oral epithelium has the following cell layers:
1. Basal layer (stratum basale or stratum germinativum).
2. Spinous layer (stratum spinosum).
3. Granular layer (stratum granulosum).
4. Keratinized cell layer (stratum corneum).

Q10. Distinguish between oral sulcular epithelium, oral epithelium and junctional epithelium.

Answer

	Junctional epithelium	Oral sulcular epithelium	Oral epithelium
Size of the cells	Large	Small	Small
Intercellular space	Wide	Narrow	Narrow
Granular layer	Absent	Absent	Present

Q11. What are the cells present in non-keratinized epithelium?

Answer

The non-keratinized epithelium contains:
1. Clear cells, which include melanocytes.
2. Langerhans cells.
3. Merkel cells and lymphocytes.

Q12. Classify gingival epithelium based on morphology and function.

Answer

1. Oral/outer epithelium: Lines the oral cavity.
2. Sulcular epithelium: Lines the gingival sulcus without being in contact with the tooth.
3. Junctional epithelium: Provides contact between the gingiva and the tooth.

Q13. What is the length of junctional epithelium?

Answer

The length of the junctional epithelium ranges from 0.25 to 1.35 mm.

Q14. What are three zones present in the junctional epithelium? What is the function of each zone?

Answer

Three zones in junctional epithelium are:
1. Apical zone for germination.
2. Middle zone for adhesion.
3. Coronal zone for permeability.

Q15. Define lamina propria and its layers.

Answer

The connective tissue supporting the oral epithelium is termed as the lamina propria and for descriptive purpose it can be divided into two layers as below:
1. *The superficial papillary layer*—associated with the epithelial ridges.
2. *Deeper reticular layer*—that lies between the papillary layer and the underlying structures.

Q16. What are the cells and fibers present in lamina propria?

Answer

Cells

Different types of cells present are:
1. Fibroblast.
2. Mast cells.
3. Macrophages.
4. Inflammatory cells.

Fibers

The connective tissue fibers are produced by fibroblasts and can be divided into:
1. Collagen fibers.
2. Reticulin fibers.
3. Oxytalan fibers.
4. Elastin fibers.

Q17. What is dentogingival unit?

Answer

The junctional epithelium and the gingival fibers are considered as a functional unit, which is also called dentogingival unit.

Q18. What are orthokeratinization, parakeratinization and non-keratinization?

Answer

Orthokeratinization: A completely keratinized epithelial layer, which is present in the superficial layer and is horny and lacks nuclei in the stratum corneum.

Parakeratinization: The stratum corneum retains the pyknotic nuclei and contains keratohyaline granules.

Non-keratinized epithelium: Does not have stratum granulosum or stratum corneum.

Q19. What is basal lamina?

Answer

Electron microscope reveals a faintly fibrillar structure called the basal lamina, which is a part of the basement membrane. This structure has lamina lucida adjacent to the basal epithelial cells and lamina densa toward connective tissue. Basal lamina is produced by adjacent epithelial cells and is made up of collagenous proteins and proteoglycans bound together into a totally-insoluble complex. It also contains laminin and fibronectin.

Q20. What are the types of keratin found in the outer epithelium?

Answer

Types of keratin found in the outer epithelium include:
1. K1, K2, K10 and K12: Expressed more in ortho-keratinized areas.
2. K6 and K16: Expressed in highly proliferative epithelia.
3. K5 and K14: Stratification specific cytokeratin.
4. K19: Usually absent from orthokeratinized epithelia.

Q21. Name the proteins synthesized by the gingival epithelium.

Answer

Proteins synthesized by epithelium include keratin, keratolinin and involucrin.

Q22. What are desmosomes and hemidesmosomes?

Answer

The cells are attached to one another by numerous desmosomes (pairs of hemidesmosomes), which are located between the cytoplasmic processes of adjacent cells.

Composition of a desmosome: It consists of two adjoining hemidesmosomes separated by a zone containing electron dense granulated material (GM).

Q23. What are odland bodies or keratinosomes?

Answer

Found in the stratum granulosum, small lamellar granules, which are glycolipid in nature. They are known as odland bodies/keratinosomes or membrane coating granules.

Q24. What are acquired and developmental coatings of the teeth?

Answer

Acquired coatings include those of exogenous origin; saliva, bacteria, calculus and surface stains.

Developmental coatings include reduced enamel epithelium, coronal cementum and dental cuticle.

Q25. What is active and passive eruption?

Answer

Active eruption is the movement of the teeth in the direction of occlusal plane.

Passive eruption is the exposure of the teeth by apical migration of gingival margin.

Q26. Enumerate gingival fibers.

Answer

The arrangement of gingival fibers is described as *principal group* of five bundles and *secondary group* of minor fibers consisting of six sets.

The principle group of fibers are:
1. Dentogingival fibers.
2. Alveolar gingival fibers.
3. Dentoperiosteal fibers.
4. Circular fibers.
5. Transseptal fibers.

Secondary group of minor fibers are:
1. Periosteogingival fibers.
2. Interpapillary fibers.
3. Transgingival fibers.
4. Intercircular fibers.
5. Intergingival fibers.
6. Semicircular fibers.

Q27. What are the functions of gingival fibers?

Answer

1. It braces the marginal gingiva firmly against the tooth.
2. It helps to withstand the forces exerted by mastication.
3. It unites the free gingiva to the root cementum and the adjacent attached gingiva.

Q28. What is blood supply of gingiva?

Answer

1. Supraperiosteal arterioles.
2. Vessels of the periodontal ligament.
3. Arterioles emerging from the crest of the interdental septa.

Q29. Enumerate lymphatic drainage and nerve supply of gingiva.

Answer

Lymphatic drainage of the gingiva brings in the lymphatics of the connective tissue papillae. It progresses to the periosteum of the alveolar process and then to regional lymph nodes (mainly submaxillary group).

Nerve supply to gingiva is derived from fibers arising from nerves in the periodontal ligament and from the labial, buccal and palatal nerves.

Q30. What is the width of periodontal ligament?

Answer

The width of periodontal ligament is approximately 0.25 mm.

Q31. What are the cells present in the periodontal ligament?

Answer

Cells of periodontal ligament are categorized as given below:
1. *Synthetic cells:*
   a. Osteoblasts.
   b. Fibroblasts.
   c. Cementoblasts.
2. *Resorptive cells:*
   a. Osteoclasts.
   b. Cementoclasts.
   c. Fibroblasts.
3. *Progenitor cells.*
4. *Other epithelial cells:* Epithelial cell rests of Malassez.
5. *Connective tissue cells like* mast cells and macrophages.

Q32. What type of collagen fibers are present in the periodontal ligament? What are they otherwise called?

Answer

The type of collagen fibers present in the periodontal ligament are mainly type I and are also called principle fibers.

Q33. What are the indifferent fiber plexus?

Answer

In the past, it was believed that in the middle portion of the periodontal ligament, there occurs splicing of fibers from cementum and bone, which forms the intermediate plexus. These plexus were thought to play a significant role in orientation and adjustment of fibers during eruption and functional movement of teeth. But recent investigations have revealed that in humans these plexus disappears once the fusion of cemental and osseous fibers are completed.

Q34. What is the principal group of fibers present in periodontal ligament?

Answer

The principal fibers in periodontal ligament include:
1. Dentogingival fibers: They project from the cementum in a fan-like conformation toward the crest and outer surface of the marginal gingiva. They provide support to the gingiva by attaching it to the tooth.
2. Alveolar gingival fibers: They extend from the periosteum of the alveolar crest coronally into the lamina propria. Their function is to attach the gingiva to the alveolar bone.
3. Dentoperiosteal fibers: They arise from the cementum near the cementoenamel junction and insert into the periosteum of the alveolar bone and protect the periodontal ligament.
4. Circular fibers: They surround the tooth in a cuff or ring-like fashion and course through the connective tissue of the marginal and attached gingiva.
5. Transseptal fibers: They are located interproximally, they extend from cementum of one tooth to the cementum of the neighboring tooth. Their function is to protect the interproximal bone and maintain tooth-to-tooth contact.

Q35. What are blood vessels supplying the periodontal ligament?

Answer

Periodontal ligament is supplied by branches derived from three sources: Dental, inter-radicular and interdental arteries.

Q36. Describe the lymphatic drainage and nerve supply of periodontal ligament.

Answer

1. Lymphatic drainage of the gingiva brings in the lymphatics of the connective tissue papillae. It progresses to the periosteum of the alveolar process and then to regional lymph nodes (mainly submaxillary group).
2. Nerve supply to gingiva is derived from fibers arising from nerves in the periodontal ligament and from the labial, buccal and palatal nerves.

Periodontal ligament is mainly supplied by the dental branches of the alveolar nerve through the apical perforations of the tooth socket or from the cribriform plate.

Q37. What are the four types of neural terminations found in the periodontal ligament?

Answer

1. Free nerve endings: Have a tree-like configuration and carry pain sensation.
2. Ruffini-like mechanoreceptors: Located primarily in the apical area.
3. Meissener's corpuscles: Also called mechano-receptors, found in mid-root region.
4. Spindle-like pressure and vibration endings: Located mainly in the apex.

Q38. What are the causes for widening of periodontal space?

Answer

The causes for widening of periodontal ligament space can be divided into the following.

Local Causes

1. Periodontitis.
2. Infection/inflammation.
3. Odontogenic tumors.
4. Trauma from occlusion.
5. Traumatic injury.
6. Iatrogenic: Excessive orthodontic forces.

Systemic Causes

1. Paget's disease.
2. Hypoparathyroidism.
3. Osteomyelitis.
4. Hypophosphatasia.
5. Scleroderma.
6. Leukemia.

Q39. What are the causes for thinning of PDL space?

Answer

Causes for thinning of PDL space are:
1. Teeth in infraocclusion.

2. Embedded teeth.
3. Physiologic aging.

Q40. What are the structures present in connective tissue?

Answer

1. Blood vessels.
2. Lymphatics.
3. Nerve innervation.
4. Cementicles.

Q41. What are the functions of periodontal ligament?

Answer

1. Physical functions.
2. Formative and remodeling functions.
3. Nutritional and sensory functions.

Q42. Define alveolar bone. What are the parts of it?

Answer

It is that portion of the maxilla and mandible that forms and supports the tooth socket (alveoli).

Alveolar bone consists of the following:
1. Inner and outer cortical plate.
2. The bone lining the socket.
3. An interior portion of cancellous bone.

Q43. What is the composition of alveolar bone?

Answer

It has two basic constituents:
1. The cells consist of osteoblasts, osteoclasts and osteocytes.
2. Extracellular matrix consists of 65% inorganic and 35% organic matter.

Q44. What is bundle bone?

Answer

Bone adjacent to periodontal ligament that contain large amount of Sharpey's fibers is called bundle bone.

Q45. What is the difference between fenestration and dehiscence?

Answer

Isolated areas in which the root is denuded of bone and the root surface is covered only by periosteum and overlying gingiva are termed fenestrations. In these areas marginal bone is intact. When the denuded areas extend through the marginal bone, the defect is called dehiscence.

Q46. Define cementum and classify it.

Answer

Cementum is a calcified avascular mesenchymal tissue that forms the outer covering of the anatomic root. It provides anchorage mainly to the principal fibers of periodontal ligament.

Depending on location, morphology and histological appearance, Schroeder and Page have classified cementum as:
1. Acellular afibrillar cementum (AAC).
2. Acellular extrinsic fiber cementum (AEFC).
3. Cellular mixed stratified cementum (CMSC).
4. Cellular intrinsic fiber cementum (CIFC).
5. Intermediate cementum (or) the hyaline layer of Hopewell-Smith.

Q47. What are the functions of cementum?

Answer

1. Primary function of cementum is to provide anchorage to the tooth in its alveolus. This is achieved through the collagen fiber bundles of the periodontal ligament, whose ends are embedded in cementum.
2. Cementum also plays an important role in maintaining occlusal relationships, whenever the incisal and occlusal surfaces are abraded due to attrition, the tooth supraerupts in order to compensate for the loss and deposition of new cementum occurs at the apical root area.

Q48. What is the composition of cementum?

Answer

The cementum is composed of both inorganic (46%) and organic matter. The organic matrix is chiefly composed of 90% type I collagen, 5% type III collagen and non-collagenous proteins like enamel proteins, adhesion molecules like tenascin and fibronectin, glycosaminoglycans like chondroitin sulfate, dermatan sulfate and heparan sulfate, which constitute the remaining organic matrix.

Q49. Enumerate the differences between acellular and cellular cementum.

Answer

Acellular Cementum

1. Forms during root.
2. Does not contain any cells.
3. Seen at the coronal portion of root.
4. Formation is slow.
5. Arrangement of collagen fibers are more organized.

Cellular Cementum

1. Forms after the eruption of the tooth and in response to functional demands.
2. Contains cementocytes.
3. Seen at a more apical portion of root.
4. Deposition is more rapid.
5. Collagen fibers are irregularly arranged.

Q50. What is hypercementosis? What is its etiology?

Answer

Hypercementosis refers to a prominent thickening of the cementum. It is largely an age-related phenomenon. It may be localized or generalized.

Causes

Local causes are excessive tension from orthodontic appliances or occlusal forces, absence of antagonist, low grade periapical irritation arising in the pulp.

Systemic causes: Neoplastic and non-neoplastic conditions including benign cementoblastoma, cementifying fibroma, periapical cemental dysplasia, florid cement-osseous dysplasia and other benign fibro-osseous lesions.

Other systemic disturbances may include acromegaly, arthritis, calcinosis, rheumatic fever and thyroid goiter.

Q51. What is intermediate cementum or hyaline layer of Hopewell-Smith?

Answer

The poorly defined zone near the cementodentinal junction of certain teeth contains cellular remnants of Hertwig's root sheath embedded in the calcified ground substance.

CHAPTER 6
Periodontal Structures in Aging Humans

Q1. What are the age changing factors on gingiva and oral mucosa?

Answer
1. Decreased keratinization.
2. Reduced or unchanged amount of stippling.
3. Decreased connective tissue cellularity.
4. Decreased oxygen consumption—which may reflect upon the metabolic activity.
5. Increased width of attached gingiva.
6. Greater amounts of intercellular substances.
7. Atrophy of the connective tissue with loss of elasticity.
8. Increase in the number of mast cells.

Q2. What changes can be seen in periodontal ligament after aging in humans?

Answer
1. Decreased vascularity.
2. Decreased mitotic activity.
3. Decrease in fibroblasts.
4. Collagen fibers and mucopolysaccharides are decreased.
5. Increase in elastic fibers and arteriosclerotic changes are seen.
6. Both increase and decrease in the width of the periodontal ligament is seen.

Q3. What are the changes that can be seen in alveolar bone and cementum in aging?

Answer
1. Osteoporosis.
2. Decreased vascularity.
3. Reduction in metabolic rate and healing capacity.
4. Resorption activity is increased and the rate of bone formation is decreased.
5. Continuous deposition of cementum occurs with age.

CHAPTER 7

Classification Systems of Periodontal Diseases

Q1. What is the need for classification?

Answer

1. For the purpose of diagnosis, prognosis and treatment planning.
2. To understand the etiology and pathology of the diseases of the periodontium.
3. For logical, systematic separation and organization of knowledge about disease.
4. Facts can be filed for future references.
5. Helps to communicate among clinicians, researchers, educators, students, epidemiologists and public health workers.

Q2. What is the classification of periodontal diseases according to World Workshop in Clinical Periodontics (1988)?

Answer

Gingivitis

1. Childhood gingivitis.
2. Chronic (adult) gingivitis.
3. Acute necrotizing ulcerative gingivitis.

Periodontitis

1. Adult periodontitis: Possible subgroups:
    a. High risk.
    b. Normal risk.
    c. Refractory periodontitis.
2. Early onset periodontitis:
    a. Localized juvenile periodontitis.
    b. Rapidly progressive periodontitis.
    c. Prepubertal periodontitis:
        i. Localized.
        ii. Generalized.
    d. Periodontitis associated with systemic diseases.

Q3. What is the classification of periodontal diseases according to World Workshop in Clinical Periodontics (1989)?

Answer

World Workshop in Clinical Periodontics (1989)

1. Adult periodontitis.
2. Early onset periodontitis:
    a. Prepubertal: Generalized or localized.
    b. Juvenile: Generalized or localized.
    c. Rapidly progressive periodontitis.
3. Periodontitis associated with systemic diseases:
    a. Down syndrome.
    b. Diabetes—Type I.
    c. Papillon-Lefévre syndrome.
    d. AIDS and other diseases.
4. Necrotizing ulcerative periodontitis.
5. Refractory periodontitis.

Q4. What are the types of chronic periodontitis?

Answer

1. Localized: Less than 30% of sites involved.
2. Generalized: More than 30% of sites involved.
3. Slight: 1–2 mm clinical attachment loss.
4. Moderate: 3–4 mm clinical attachment loss.
5. Severe: More than 5 mm clinical attachment loss.

Q5. What are the types of aggressive periodontitis?

Answer

Based on distribution:
1. Localized: Less than 30% of sites involved.
2. Generalized: More than 30% of sites involved.

Based on disease severity:
1. Slight: 1–2 mm clinical attachment loss.
2. Moderate: 3–4 mm clinical attachment loss.
3. Severe: More than 5 mm clinical attachment loss.

Q6. What are the manifestations of systemic diseases in periodontitis?

Answer
1. Associated with hematological disorders:
    a. Acquired neutropenia.
    b. Leukemias.
    c. Others.
2. Associated with genetic disorders:
    a. Familial and cyclic neutropenia.
    b. Down syndrome.
    c. Leukocyte adhesion deficiency syndrome.
    d. Papillon-Lefévre syndrome.
    e. Chediak-Higashi syndrome.
    f. Histiocytosis syndrome.
    g. Glycogen storage disease.
    h. Infantile genetic agranulocytosis.
    i. Cohen syndrome.
    j. Ehlers-Danlos syndrome (Types IV and VIII).
    k. Hypophosphatasia.
    l. Others.

CHAPTER 8
Epidemiology of Gingival and Periodontal Diseases

Q1. Define epidemiology.

Answer

Study of health and disease in populations and how the states are influenced by heredity, biology, physical and social environmental ways of living.

Q2. What are the types of epidemiological research?

Answer

1. Descriptive studies.
2. Analytical studies.
3. Experimental epidemiology.

Q3. What is incidence rate?

Answer

Incidence rate is defined as the number of new cases occurring in a defined population during a specific period of time.

Q4. What is prevalence rate? What are the types of prevalence?

Answer

Prevalence rate refers to all current cases (new and old) existing at a given point of time or over a period of time in a given population. Two types are described as follows:
1. Point prevalence.
2. Period prevalence.

Q5. What is longitudinal study? What are its uses?

Answer

In longitudinal study, the observations are repeated in the same population over a prolonged period of time by means of follow-up examinations.

Uses

1. To study the natural history of disease and its future outcome.
2. For identifying the risk factors of disease.
3. For finding out the incidence rate or rate of occurrence of new cases.

Q6. What is cross-sectional study? What are its uses?

Answer

It is the simplest form of an observational study. It is based on a single examination of a cross-section of population at one point of time (it is also known as prevalence study).

Uses

1. It is more useful for chronic (long-term diseases) as compared to acute (short-term) diseases.
2. It gives information about the distribution of a disease in a population rather than its etiology.

Q7. What are the types of analytical study?

Answer

It includes two distinct types as given below:
1. Case-control study.
2. Cohort study.

Q8. Define index. What are the purposes of it?

Answer

These are numerical values describing the relative status of the population on a graduated scale with definite upper and lower limits, which are designed to permit and facilitate comparisons with other populations.

For Individual Patients

An index can:
1. Provide individual assessment to help a patient to recognize an oral problem.
2. Reveal the degree of effectiveness of present oral hygiene practices.

In Research

An index is used to:
1. Determine the baseline data before the experimental factors are introduced.
2. Measure the effectiveness of specific agents for the prevention, control and treatment of oral conditions.
3. Measures the effectiveness of mechanical devices for personal care such as toothbrushes, interdental cleaning devices or water irrigators.

Q9. Mention some indices used in periodontal destruction.

Answer

1. Russell's periodontal index.
2. Periodontal disease index (PDI) by Ramfjord.
3. Extent and severity index by Carlos and coworkers.
4. Radiographic approaches to measure bone loss:
    a. Gingival bone count index (GBI) by Dunning and Leach.
    b. Periodontal severity index (PSI) by Adams and Nystrom.

Q10. Enumerate various indices used to measure plaque accumulation.

Answer

Indices Used to Measure Plaque Accumulation

1. Plaque component of periodontal disease index by Ramfjord.
2. Simplified oral hygiene index by Greene and Vermillion.
3. Turesky-Gilmore-Glickman modification of the Quigley-Hein plaque index.
4. Plaque index by Silness and Loe.
5. Modified navy plaque index.
6. Patient hygiene performance (PHP) index by Podshadley and Haley.
7. Plaque weight.
8. Plaque free score by Grant, Stern and Everett.
9. Plaque control record by O'Leary.

Q11. What are the indices used to measure calculus?

Answer

Indices Used to Measure Calculus

1. Calculus component of simplified oral hygiene index by Greene and Vermillion.
2. Calculus component of the periodontal disease index by Ramfjord.
3. Probe method of calculus assessment by Volpe and associates.
4. Calculus surface index by Ennever and coworkers.
5. Marginal line calculus index by Mühlemann and Villa.

Q12. What are the indices used to measure gingival inflammation?

Answer

1. Papillary marginal attached (PMA) index by Schour and Massler.
2. Gingivitis component of the periodontal disease.
3. Gingival index by Loe and Silness.
4. Indices for gingival bleeding:
    a. Sulcus bleeding index (SBI) of Mühlemann and Mazor.
    b. Papillary bleeding index (PBI) by Mühlemann.
    c. Bleeding points index by Lennox and Kopczyk.
    d. Interdental bleeding index by Caton and Polson.
    e. Gingival bleeding index by Ainamo and Bay.

Q13. What are indices used to assess treatment needs?

Answer

1. Gingival periodontal index.
2. Community periodontal index of treatment needs by Ainamo and associates.
3. Periodontal treatment need system (PTNS) by Belini HT.

Q14. Who has given gingival index?

Answer

Loe and Silness.

Q15. Who has given plaque index?

Answer

Silness and Loe.

Q16. What are the scoring criteria for simplified oral hygiene index?

Answer

Simplified oral hygiene index has two parts as mentioned below:
1. Debris index-simplified (DI-S).
2. Calculus index-simplified (CI-S).

Scoring Criteria for DI-S

0: No debris or stain present.
1: Soft debris covering not more than one-third of the tooth surface or the presence of extrinsic stains without other debris, regardless of surface area covered.
2: Soft debris covering more than one-third, but not more than two-thirds of the exposed tooth surface.

3: Soft debris covering more than two-thirds of the exposed tooth surface.

Scoring Criteria for CI-S

0: No calculus present.
1: Supragingival calculus covering not more than one-third of the exposed tooth surface.
2: Supragingival calculus covering more than one-third, but not more than two-thirds of the exposed tooth surface or the presence of the individual flecks of subgingival calculus around the cervical portion of the tooth or both.
3: Supragingival calculus covering more than two-thirds of the exposed tooth surface or a continuous heavy band of subgingival calculus around the cervical portion of the tooth or both.

Q17. What are the scoring criteria for plaque index (Silness and Loe)?

Answer

Scoring Criteria

0: No plaque in the gingival area.
1: A film of plaque adhering to the free gingival margin and adjacent area of the tooth. The plaque may be recognized only by running a probe across the tooth surface.
2: Moderate accumulation of soft deposits within the gingival pocket and on the gingival margin and/or adjacent tooth surface that can be seen by naked eye.
3: Abundance of soft matter within the gingival pocket and/or on the gingival margin and adjacent tooth surface.

CHAPTER 9

Periodontal Microbiology

Q1. Define dental plaque.

Answer

Dental plaque is an adherent intercellular matrix consisting primarily of proliferating microorganisms, along with a scattering of epithelial cells, leukocytes and macrophages.

Q2. Define biofilm.

Answer

Biofilms are defined as matrix-enclosed bacterial populations adherent to each other and/or to surface or interfaces (Costerton). According to the recent data (Widerer and Charaklis, 1989), biofilm is defined as the relatively undefinable microbial community associated with a tooth surface or any other hard, non-shedding material.

Q3. What are the salient features of biofilm?

Answer

1. Ability to trap and concentrate the nutrients required for the growth of microorganisms.
2. Involved in the metabolism of their own nutrients.
3. Resistant to host defenses.
4. Protects the bacteria in the biofilm from antibiotics and antimicrobials.

Q4. What are the types of dental plaque?

Answer

Based on its relationship to the gingival margin, plaque is differentiated into two categories, supragingival and subgingival plaque.

Supragingival plaque is further differentiated into: Coronal plaque, which is in contact with only the tooth surface and marginal plaque, which is associated with tooth surface at the gingival margin.

Subgingival plaque can be further differentiated into:
1. Attached plaque.
2. Unattached subgingival plaque.
3. Attached plaque can be tooth, epithelium and/or connective tissue associated.

Q5. Mention bacterial flora caused by tooth-associated subgingival plaque.

Answer

The flora is dominated by gram-positive cocci, rods, filamentous bacteria and some/few gram-negative cocci and rods. This flora is associated with calculus formation, root caries and root resorption.

Q6. What is the composition of plaque?

Answer

Bacteria + intercellular matrix = dental plaque

Intercellular matrix is composed of organic and inorganic constituents, which are derived from saliva, gingival crevicular fluid (GCF) and bacterial products.

Q7. What are the factors influencing rate of plaque formation?

Answer

Factors influencing rate of plaque formation include the following:
1. Surface microroughness.
2. Oral hygiene status.
3. Diet.
4. Chewing fibrous food.
5. Smoking.
6. Tongue and palate brushing.
7. Colloid stability of the bacteria in the saliva.
8. Antimicrobial factors present in the saliva.
9. Chemical composition of the pellicle.
10. Retention depth of the dentogingival area.

Q8. What is co-aggregation?

Answer

The process by which different species and genera of plaque microorganisms adhere to one another is called co-aggregation.

Q9. What are the different types of bacterial complexes?

Answer

Based on the frequency of clustering, Socransky classified microorganisms into different complexes:

Yellow complex: *Streptococcus.*
Purple complex: *Actinomyces odontolyticus.*
Green complex: *Eikenella corrodens, Actinobacillus actinomycetemcomitans* serotype a and *Capnocytophaga* species.
Orange complex: *Fusobacterium, Prevotella, Campylobacter* species.
Red complex: *Porphyromonas gingivalis, Tannerella forsythia, Treponema denticola.*

Q10. Describe the formation of dental plaque.

Answer

Plaque formation occurs in the following stages:
1st stage: Pellicle formation induces absorption of salivary proteins to appetite surfaces.
2nd stage: Initial colonization of the tooth surface by primary colonizers like *Actinomyces viscosus* and *Streptococcus* species *(Streptococcus sanguinis).*
3rd stage: Secondary colonization and plaque maturation: Secondary colonizers are *Prevotella intermedia, Capnocytophaga, Porphyromonas gingivalis, Fusobacterium nucleatum.*

Q11. What is the clinical significance of plaque?

Answer

The microbial aggregations on the tooth surface if prevented from maturing may become compatible with gingival health. Supragingival plaque if allowed to grow and mature may induce gingivitis and can lead to the formation of a microenvironment that permits the development of subgingival plaque. Therefore, supragingival plaque is pathogenic. According to this, when only small amounts of plaque are present, the products released by this get neutralized by the host. Similarly, large amounts of plaque would produce large amounts of noxious products, which would overwhelm the host's defenses. However, several authors have contradicted this concept. First, many patients have considerable amounts of plaque and calculus as well as gingivitis, but only a minority suffer from destructive periodontal disease even then in only few sites.

Q12. Describe specific plaque hypothesis.

Answer

Specific plaque hypothesis, which states that destructive periodontal disease, is a result of specific microbial pathogens in plaque. Thus, although the amount of plaque present correlates well with disease severity, it correlates poorly in individual patients.

Q13. Describe non-specific plaque hypothesis.

Answer

Non-specific plaque hypothesis, which forms the basis for virtually all the current modalities of treatment and prevention, which relies on the principle of reducing plaque scores to a minimum. Thus, although the non-specific plaque hypothesis has been discarded in favor of the specific plaque hypothesis, much clinical treatment is still based on the non-specific plaque hypothesis.

Q14. What makes the plaque pathogenic?

Answer

The following are the possible pathogenic mechanisms by which the plaque microorganisms can cause periodontal disease:
1. Physical nature of plaque.
2. Invasion of tissues by bacteria.
3. Release of toxic and inflammatory substances.
4. Role of bacterial specificity.

CHAPTER 10

Calculus and Other Etiological Factors

Q1. Define calculus.

Answer

Dental calculus is an adherent, calcified or calcifying mass that forms on the surfaces of teeth and dental appliances. It is covered on its external surface by vital, tightly adherent, non-mineralized plaque.

Q2. What are the types of calculus?

Answer

Depending upon the position of calculus in relation to the marginal gingiva it is classified as:
1. Supragingival calculus.
2. Subgingival calculus.

Q3. What is the composition of calculus?

Answer

Inorganic components	Dry weight (in %)
Calcium	27–29
Phosphorus	16–18
Carbonate	2–3
Sodium	1.5–2.5
Magnesium	0.6–0.8
Fluoride	0.003–0.04
Crystal forms	
Hydroxyapatite	58
Magnesium whitlockite	21
Octacalcium phosphate	12
Brushite	9
Organic components	Dry weight (in %)
Mixture of protein, polysaccharide complexes, desquamated epithelial cells, leukocytes and various microorganisms; carbohydrate (consists of glucose, galactose, rhamnose, mannose)	1.9–9.1
Proteins	5.9–8.2
Lipids	0.2

Q4. What are the major crystal forms seen in the inorganic component of calculus?

Answer

The major crystal forms include the following:
1. Hydroxyapatite.
2. Magnesium whitlockite.
3. Octacalcium phosphate.
4. Brushite.

Q5. Describe the formation of calculus.

Answer

Calculus is dental plaque that has undergone mineralization. Calculus is formed by the precipitation of mineral salts, which can start between 1st and 14th day of plaque formation. In two days, plaque can be 50% mineralized and 60%–90% gets mineralized in 12 days. Calcification starts in separate foci on the inner surface of the plaque. These foci of mineralization gradually increase in size and coalesce to form a solid mass of calculus.

Q6. What is calculocementum?

Answer

Calculus embedded deeply in cementum may appear morphologically similar to cementum and thus has been termed calculocementum.

Q7. What is the time required for plaque to get mineralized?

Answer

Calcification of plaque occurs as soon as 4–8 hours. Calcifying plaque may become 50% mineralized in 2 days and 60%–90% mineralized in 12 days.

Q8. What are the theories of calculus formation?

Answer

It can be explained mainly under the following categories:
1. Precipitation of minerals can occur from a local rise in the degree of saturation of calcium and phosphate ions, this is explained in the following:

a. *Booster mechanism.*
b. *Colloidal proteins* in saliva bind to calcium and phosphate ions thus producing a super-saturated solution.
c. *Phosphatase* liberated from dental plaque, desquamated epithelial cells or bacteria precipitate calcium phosphate by hydrolyzing organic phosphates in saliva.
2. Another concept that has been most widely held is 'Epitactic concept' (heterogenous nucleation).
3. Inhibition theory.

Q9. What are differences between supragingival and subgingival calculus?

Answer

Supragingival calculus	Subgingival calculus
Location—above the gingival margin	Deposits present below the gingival margin
Color—white, yellow in color	Brown or greenish black
Source—derived from salivary secretions	Formed from gingival exudate
Composition—more brushite and octacalcium phosphate less magnesium whitlockite	Conversely less brushite and octacalcium phosphate and more magnesium whitlockite
Salivary proteins are present	Salivary proteins are absent
Sodium content is lesser	Sodium content increases with the depth of the pocket

Q10. What is the clinical significance of calculus?

Answer

It mostly contributes to gingival inflammation and periodontal disease by providing a base for non-mineralized plaque, which is the main etiologic factor for periodontal disease. Hence, calculus acts only as a contributing factor for periodontal disease.

Q11. What is material alba?

Answer

It is a yellow, grayish white, soft sticky deposit consisting of cells, neutrophils, salivary proteins, lipid with little or no food particles. They lack internal structure seen in plaque, hence can be easily washed away with water spray.

Q12. What are plunger cusps?

Answer

Cusps that tend to forcibly wedge food interproximally are known as 'Plunger cusps'.

Q13. What are the causes of food impaction?

Answer

1. Uneven occlusal wear.
2. Loss of proximal contact.
3. Congenital, morphologic abnormalities of teeth.
4. Improperly-constructed restorations.
5. Lateral food impaction.

Q14. What are the sequelae following food impaction?

Answer

1. Feeling of pressure and urge to dig the material from between the teeth.
2. The premolars move distally and the mandibular incisors tilt or drift lingually.
3. The anterior overbite is increased. The mandibular incisors strike the maxillary incisors near the gingiva or traumatize the gingiva.
4. The maxillary incisors are pushed labially and laterally.
5. The anterior teeth extrude, because the incisal opposition has largely disappeared.
6. Diastema is created by the separation of the anterior teeth.

Q15. Explain about stains.

Answer

Pigmented deposits on tooth surface are called stains. Discoloration of teeth can occur in three different ways as given below:
1. Stains adhering directly to tooth surface.
2. Stains contained within the calculus and soft deposits.
3. Stains incorporated within the tooth structure or restorative material.

Q16. What is the classification of stains?

Answer

Based on Location
1. Extrinsic stains.
2. Intrinsic stains.

Based on Source
1. Exogenous.
2. Endogenous.

Q17. Mention some extrinsic stains.

Answer

1. Tobacco stain.
2. Black stain.

3. Green stain.
4. Orange stain.
5. Metallic stain.
6. Chlorhexidine stain.

Q18. Mention some intrinsic stains.

Answer

1. *Exogenous sources:*
   a. Restorative materials.
   b. Drugs.
2. *Endogenous sources:* For example, non-vital tooth:
   a. Developmental anomalies namely amelogenesis imperfecta, dentinogenesis imperfecta.
   b. Enamel hypoplasia.
   c. Dental fluorosis.
   d. Erythroblastosis fetalis.

Q19. What is Sorrin's classification of habits?

Answer

1. Neuroses: Lip biting, cheek biting, occlusal neuroses like bruxism and clenching.
2. Occupational habits: Like cobblers/carpenters holding nails between the teeth.
3. Miscellaneous habits: Smoking, mouth breathing, thumb sucking and improper toothbrushing.

CHAPTER 11

Host Response: Basic Concepts

Q1. What is GCF? What are its functions?
Answer

Gingival crevicular fluid (GCF) is the fluid, which is found in the gingival sulcus. Its main functions are:
1. Washing non-adherent bacteria and their products out of the crevice.
2. Reducing the diffusion of plaque products into the tissues.
3. It also carries a steady supply of inflammatory mediators, protease inhibitors and host defense agents such as complement and antibodies into the crevice.

Q2. What is complement system?
Answer

It is a system of series of non-specific proteins present in normal human and animal serum, which are activated by antigen-antibody reaction and subsequently lead to biologically significant consequences such as cell lysis or damage of target cells.

Q3. What is the sequence of classical pathway?
Answer

Classical pathway
C1 → C4 → C2 → C3 → C5 → C6 → C7 → C8 → C9

Q4. What is the sequence of alternative pathway?
Answer

Alternative pathway
C3 → C5 → C6 → C7 → C8 → C9

Q5. Explain the terms rolling and margination in terms of neutrophils. Also describe diapedesis/interendothelial transmigration.
Answer

Leukocytes normally travel along the center of the lumen of the blood vessel, but in inflamed tissues the blood flow is slowed by fluid exudation and they adhere more readily to endothelial cells. This mechanism is called rolling and margination.

When the neutrophils migrate across the endothelium it is called diapedesis and interendothelial transmigration.

Q6. What is the role of macrophages in development of host response?
Answer

Macrophages develop from blood monocytes, which emigrate into the tissues from the blood and are triggered to develop into mature macrophages by cytokines, other inflammatory mediators and bacterial products such as endotoxins. Functions of macrophages include:
1. Phagocytose and kill bacteria.
2. Remove damaged host tissue during inflammation.
3. Trap and present antigens to lymphocytes for induction of immune responses.

Since these functions unite inflammation and immunity, the macrophages play an important role in all bacterial infections and hence help in developing host response against pathogenic infections.

Q7. What are the different stages in neutrophil chemotaxis?
Answer

Stage 1: Formation of concentration gradient.
Stage 2: Detection of chemotaxins by neutrophils.
Stage 3: Polarization of neutrophils.
Stage 4: Neutrophils crawl up to concentration gradient.
Stage 5: Directional migration ceases after concentration is constant.

Q8. What is opsonization?
Answer

For efficient phagocytosis, the particle should be coated with one or more host serum proteins. This process is

called opsonization. Two principal types of serum proteins referred as opsonins are:
- IgG
- C3b.

Opsonization could be complement dependent, antibody dependent or combination of both.

Q9. What are the various killing mechanisms activated during phagocytosis?

Answer

1. Oxygen-dependent killing mechanism: Stimulation by phagocytic cells increase the cellular consumption of oxygen called respiratory burst. Majority of oxygen consumed by phagocytes are converted into superoxide ion through action of NADPH oxidase. This in turn undergoes conversion into H_2O_2, which contributes to microbial activity of phagocytes.

    Additionally hypochlorous acid and toxic aldehydes are also produced. Oxygen-dependent bactericidal action could be myeloperoxidase dependent or independent.
2. Non-oxidative mechanism: It is based on various components of cells.

Neutrophils contain three types of granules:
1. Primary/Azurophilic granules: Myeloperoxidase, lysozyme, acid phosphatase and acid hydrolases.
2. Secondary/Specific granules: Lactoferrin, lysozyme, azurocidin.
3. Tertiary granules: Alkaline phosphatase, collagenase and gelatinase.

Q10. What are the various disorders associated with periodontal diseases?

Answer

1. Diabetes mellitus.
2. Papillon-Lefevre syndrome.
3. Down syndrome.
4. Chediak-Higashi syndrome.
5. Drug-induced agranulocytosis.
6. Cyclic neutropenia.

Q11. What are the various periodontal diseases associated with neutrophil disorders?

Answer

1. Acute necrotizing ulcerative gingivitis.
2. Localized juvenile periodontitis.
3. Prepubertal periodontitis.
4. Rapidly progressive periodontitis.
5. Refractory periodontitis.

Q12. Which immune cells play an important role in acute infection?

Answer

Neutrophils.

Q13. Which immune cells play an important role in chronic infections?

Answer

Lymphocytes and macrophages.

Q14. What are the contents of specific granules?

Answer

Lysozyme and lactoferrin.

Q15. What are the contents of azurophilic granules?

Answer

Cathepsin G, α-defensins and lysozyme.

CHAPTER 12

Trauma from Occlusion

Q1. What is trauma from occlusion?
Answer

When occlusal forces exceed the adaptive capacity of periodontal tissues, these result in tissue injury. This injury is trauma from occlusion (TFO).

The WHO defined TFO as damage in the periodontium caused by the stress on teeth produced directly or indirectly by the teeth of opposite jaw.

Q2. Classify TFO.
Answer

Trauma from occlusion can be classified as:
1. Depending upon onset of duration, i.e. acute TFO and chronic TFO.
2. Depending upon the cause, i.e. primary TFO and secondary TFO.

Q3. What is the difference between primary and secondary TFO?
Answer

Primary TFO occurs due to the trauma to normal periodontium with normal height. The adaptive capacity of the periodontium is not reduced, but rather the magnitude of force increases beyond the limits of adaptability. Secondary TFO occurs when the adaptive capacity of the periodontium is reduced, e.g. in periodontitis.

Q4. What are the clinical signs and symptoms of TFO?
Answer

Clinical signs are:
1. Acute situations: Excessive tooth pain, tenderness on percussion, increased tooth mobility, formation of periodontal abscess, cemental tears, infrabony pockets, furcation involvement, attrition, pathologic migration.
2. Fremitus test is positive.

Q5. What are the radiographic changes seen in TFO?
Answer

These are:
1. Increase in width of periodontal ligament space often with thickening of lamina dura along the lateral borders of the root, apical and bifurcation areas.
2. Vertical bone loss.
3. Radiolucency and condensation of the alveolar bone.
4. Root resorption.

Q6. What is the response of periodontal tissues toward increased occlusal forces?
Answer

The response of the periodontal tissue is stagewise as following.

Stage 1: Injury

When a tooth is exposed to excessive occlusal forces, the periodontal tissues are unable to withstand and hence they distribute, while maintaining the stability of the tooth. This may lead to certain well-defined reactions in the periodontal ligament and alveolar bone. The injury phase shows an increase in areas of resorption and a decrease in bone formation.

Stage 2: Repair

The TFO stimulates increased reparative activity. When bone is resorbed by excessive occlusal forces, the body attempts to reinforce the thinned bony trabeculae with new bone. This attempt to compensate for lost bone is called buttressing bone formation, which is an important feature of reparative process associated with TFO.

The repair phase shows increase in areas of bone formation and decreased resorption.

Stage 3: Adaptive Remodeling of the Periodontium

If the repair process cannot keep pace with the destruction caused by occlusion, the periodontium may get remodeled in order to maintain the structural relationship. This may result in thickened periodontal ligament, angular defects in the bone with no pocket formation, loose teeth and increased vascularization.

Remodeling phase shows return of normal resorption and formation.

Q7. What is the effect of insufficient occlusal forces on periodontium?

Answer

It may also be injurious to periodontal tissues, which results in the thinning of the periodontal ligament, atrophy of the fibers, osteoporosis of alveolar bone and reduction in alveolar bone height. Hypofunction can result from an open bite relationship, absence of functional antagonists or unilateral chewing habits.

Q8. Is TFO reversible or irreversible?

Answer

Trauma from occlusion is reversible. When the injurious force is removed, the repair occurs. The presence of inflammation in the periodontium as a result of plaque accumulation may impair the reversibility of traumatic lesions.

Q9. What is the role of TFO in progression of periodontal diseases?

Answer

In Glickman's concept, he claimed that the pathway of the spread of plaque associated gingival lesion can be changed if the forces of an abnormal magnitude are acting on teeth harboring subgingival plaque. Teeth, which are non-traumatized, exhibit suprabony pockets and horizontal bone loss, whereas teeth with trauma exhibit angular bony defects and infrabony pockets.

Q10. What happens when a tooth with gingival inflammation is exposed to trauma?

Answer

Four possibilities can occur when a tooth with gingival inflammation is exposed to trauma:
1. Trauma from occlusion may alter the pathway of extension of gingival inflammation to the underlying tissues. Inflammation may proceed to the periodontal ligament rather than to the alveolar bone and the resulting bone loss would be angular with infrabony pockets.
2. It may favor the environment for the formation and attachment of plaque and calculus. It may be responsible for development of deeper lesions.
3. Supragingival plaque can become subgingival if the tooth is tilted orthodontically or migrates into an edentulous area, resulting in the transformation of a suprabony pocket into an infrabony pocket.
4. Increased tooth mobility associated with trauma to the periodontium may have a pumping effect on plaque metabolites increasing their diffusion.

Q11. What is pathologic tooth migration?

Answer

It refers to tooth displacement that results when the balance among the factors that maintain physiologic tooth position is disturbed by periodontal disease.

Q12. What is the pathogenesis of pathologic tooth migration?

Answer

Two major factors play a role in maintaining the normal position of the teeth:
1. The health and normal height of the periodontium: A tooth with weakened periodontal support is unable to withstand the forces and moves away from the opposing force.
2. The forces exerted on the teeth: Changes in the forces may occur as a result of:
   a. Unreplaced missing teeth.
   b. Failure to replace first molars.
   c. Other causes.

Q13. What is the role of unreplaced missing tooth in pathologic tooth migration?

Answer

This leads to drifting of teeth into the spaces created by unreplaced missing teeth. It usually creates conditions that lead to periodontal diseases and thus the initial tooth movement is aggravated by loss of periodontal support.

Q14. What is the difference between drifting and pathological tooth migration?

Answer

Drifting differs from pathologic migration in that it does not result from destruction of the periodontal tissues.

Q15. What is the pathogenesis of not replacing a missing first molar?

Answer

It consists of the following:
1. The second and third molars tilt resulting in decrease in vertical dimension.
2. The premolars move distally and the mandibular incisors tilt or drift lingually.

3. Anterior overbite is increased.
4. The maxillary incisors are pushed labially and laterally.
5. The anterior teeth extrude due to disappearance of incisal apposition.
6. Diastema is created by the separation of the anterior teeth.

Q16. Does TFO has any effect on supracrestal gingival fibers?
Answer: No.

Q17. Can unilateral or jiggling forces result in pocket formation?
Answer: No.

CHAPTER 13
Role of Systemic Diseases in the Etiology of Periodontal Diseases

Q1. What is the relationship between ascorbic acid and periodontal diseases?

Answer

1. Low levels of ascorbic acid influences the metabolism of collagen within the periodontium, thereby affecting the ability of the tissue to regenerate and repair by itself.
2. It interferes with bone formation leading to the loss of the alveolar bone.
3. Increases the permeability of oral mucosa to tritiated endotoxin and inulin.
4. Increased levels of ascorbic acid enhance both the chemotactic and migratory action of leukocytes without influencing phagocytic activity.
5. Optimal level of ascorbic acid is required to maintain the integrity of the periodontal microvasculature as well as the vascular response to bacterial irritation and wound healing.
6. Depletion of vitamin C may interfere with the ecologic equilibrium of bacteria in plaque and increases its pathogenicity.

Q2. What are the periodontal features of scurvy?

Answer

The oral symptoms are that of chronic gingivitis, which can involve the free gingiva, attached gingiva and alveolar mucosa. In severe cases, the gingiva becomes brilliant red, tender and grossly swollen. The spongy tissues are extremely hyperemic and bleed spontaneously. In long standing cases, the tissues attain a dark blue or purple hue. Alveolar bone resorption with increased tooth mobility has also been reported.

Q3. What are the radiographic findings involving periodontium in vitamin D deficiency?

Answer

There is a generalized partial-to-complete disappearance of the lamina dura and reduced density of supporting bone, loss of trabeculae, increased radiolucency of the trabecular interstices and increased prominence of the remaining trabeculae.

Q4. What is the role of deficiency of vitamin B complex in oral diseases?

Answer

Oral disease is rarely due to a deficiency in just one component of the B-complex group. Oral changes common to vitamin B-complex deficiencies are gingivitis, glossitis, glossodynia, angular cheilitis and inflammation of the entire oral mucosa.

Q5. Which are the different types of white blood cell (WBC) disorders that affect periodontium?

Answer

Disorders of WBC can be of two types:
1. Quantitative: These are neutropenia, leukemia, thrombocytopenic purpura.
2. Qualitative: These are Chédiak-Higashi syndrome, lazy leukocyte syndrome, chronic granulomatous disease.

Q6. What are the different types of neutropenia?

Answer

1. Cyclic neutropenia.
2. Chronic benign neutropenia of childhood.
3. Benign familial neutropenia.
4. Severe familial neutropenia.
5. Chronic idiopathic neutropenia.

Q7. What is cyclic neutropenia? What are its effects on periodontium?

Answer

It is characterized by a cyclic depression of the polymorphonuclear neutrophil (PMN) count in peripheral blood. The cyclic intervals are usually between 19 and 21 days. Clinical problems include pyrexia, oral ulceration and skin infections.

Periodontal manifestations: These include oral ulceration, inflamed gingiva, rapid periodontal breakdown, and alveolar bone loss. Bone loss is most obvious around the lower incisors and first permanent molars.

Treatment: Plaque control, supportive measures like antiseptic mouth wash, antimicrobial therapy, etc. has been proposed.

Q8. What are the periodontal features of chronic benign neutropenia of childhood?

Answer

The onset is usually between 6 and 20 months of age and in most patients, the condition is self-limiting. The main periodontal feature is a bright-red, hyperplastic, edematous gingiva confined to the width of attached gingiva. The gingival tissues exhibit bleeding on probing and show areas of desquamation, varying degrees of gingival recession and pocketing.

Q9. What are the periodontal features of benign familial neutropenia?

Answer

The periodontal manifestations include hyperplastic gingivitis exhibiting edematous and bright-red appearance. There is marked bone loss around the first molars. The gingival tissues bleed profusely on probing.

Q10. What is leukemia?

Answer

It is a malignant disease caused by proliferation of WBC forming tissue, especially those in bone marrow.

Q11. What are the periodontal manifestations of leukemia?

Answer

The major manifestations are gingival enlargement, gingival bleeding and periodontal infections. The incidence and severity of these problems vary according to the type and nature of leukemia.

Q12. What is the treatment plan for leukemic patients?

Answer

Treatment Plan for Leukemic Patients

1. Refer the patient for medical evaluation and treatment.
2. Prior to chemotherapy, a complete periodontal plan should be developed:
   a. Monitor hematologic laboratory values.
   b. Administer suitable antibiotics before any periodontal treatment.
   c. Periodontal treatment consists of scaling and root planing; twice daily rinsing with 0.12% chlorhexidine gluconate is recommended. If there is irregular bleeding time, careful debridement with cotton pellets soaked in 3% hydrogen peroxide is performed.

Q13. What are the clinical manifestations and treatment plan for thrombocytopenic purpura?

Answer

Clinical Manifestations

Clinical manifestations include spontaneous bleeding into skin or from mucous membranes. Petechiae and hemorrhagic vesicles occur in the oral cavity. Gingiva is swollen, soft and friable. Bleeding occurs spontaneously.

Treatment

1. Physician referral for a definitive diagnosis.
2. Oral hygiene instructions.
3. Prophylactic treatment of potential abscesses.
4. No surgical procedures are indicated unless platelet count is at least 80,000 cells/mm^3.
5. Scaling and root planing may be carefully performed at low platelet levels.

If surgery is indicated, it should be as atraumatic as possible, stents or thrombin-soaked cotton pellets placed interproximally, gentle hydrogen peroxide mouth washes and close postsurgical follow-up is recommended.

Q14. Describe the effect of qualitative disorders of WBC on periodontium.

Answer

Chédiak-Higashi Syndrome

Severe gingival inflammation appears to be a common finding in Chédiak-Higashi syndrome. The nature of the inflammatory changes may be plaque induced, secondary to infection or related to the underlying polymorphonuclear leukocyte's (PMNL's) defect.

Lazy Leukocyte Syndrome

The feature of the syndrome is a defect in leukocyte chemotaxis and random mobility. Marked gingivitis has also been described.

Chronic Granulomatous Disease

Periodontal manifestations include marked, diffuse, gingivitis with an accompanying ulceration of buccal mucosa.

Q15. What are the various red blood cell (RBC) disorders affecting periodontium?

Answer

1. Aplastic anemia.

2. Fanconi's anemia.
3. Sickle cell anemia.
4. Acatalasia.

Q16. Describe the effect of Fanconi's anemia on periodontal tissues.

Answer

This is a rare type of aplastic anemia characterized by a familial bone marrow hypoplasia that becomes manifested in the 1st decade of life. The periodontal manifestations being loss of several teeth, severe bone loss with pocketing greater than 10 mm. The gingiva will be bluish red, bleed on probing and shows suppuration on gentle pressure.

Q17. What is the association between diabetes mellitus and periodontitis?

Answer

Diabetic patient is more susceptible to periodontal breakdown, which is characterized by extensive bone loss, increased tooth mobility, widening of periodontal ligament space, suppuration and abscess formation.

Q18. What is the treatment plan for periodontal treatment in diabetes mellitus patients?

Answer

1. Periodontal treatment in patient with uncontrolled diabetes is contraindicated.
2. If suspected to be a diabetic, following procedures should be performed:
    a. Consult the patient's physician.
    b. Analyze laboratory tests, fasting blood glucose, postprandial blood glucose, glycated hemoglobin, glucose tolerance test (GTT), urinary glucose.
    c. If there is periodontal condition that requires immediate care, prophylactic antibiotics should be given.
    d. If patient is a 'brittle' diabetic, optimal periodontal health is a necessity. Glucose levels should be continuously monitored and periodontal treatment should be performed when the disease is in a well-controlled state. Prophylactic antibiotics should be started 2 days preoperatively; penicillin is the drug of first choice.

Q19. What is the effect of hyperparathyroidism on periodontal tissues?

Answer

There is:
1. Generalized demineralization of bone.
2. Tooth mobility.
3. Malocclusion.
4. Radiographic evidence of alveolar osteoporosis, widening of periodontal space and absence of lamina dura.

Q20. What are the changes, which occur in gingiva during pregnancy?

Answer

1. Pronounced base of bleeding.
2. Gingiva is bright red to bluish red.
3. Marginal and interdental gingiva is edematous, pits on pressure and sometimes presents raspberry-like appearance.
4. There is depression of maternal T-lymphocyte response.
5. Increased levels of progesterone hormone, which produce dilatation and tortuosity of the gingival microvasculature, circulatory stasis and increased susceptibility to mechanical irritation.

Q21. What is the treatment plan for gingival diseases during pregnancy?

Answer

Elimination of all local irritants that are responsible for precipitating gingival changes. Marginal and interdental gingival inflammation and enlargement are treated with scaling and root planing. Treatment of tumor-like gingival enlargements consists of surgical excision, scaling and planing of tooth surfaces.

In pregnancy emphasis should be on:
1. Preventing gingival disease before it occurs.
2. Treating existing gingival disease before it becomes worse.

Q22. What is the clinical management of periodontal diseases in breastfeeding patients?

Answer

In breastfeeding patients, certain drugs should not be prescribed as these drugs can pass into child via milk. These drugs have low safety tolerance in children. These drugs to be avoided are tetracycline, metronidazole, ciprofloxacin, Aspirin and barbiturates.

If needed, amoxicillin can be prescribed with instruction that it should be taken just after breastfeeding and then avoided for 4 hours or more.

CHAPTER 14

Oral Malodor

Q1. What are the causes of physiologic halitosis?
Answer

1. Mouth breathing.
2. Medications.
3. Aging and poor dental hygiene.
4. Fasting/starvation.
5. Tobacco.
6. Foods (onion, garlic, etc.) and alcohol.

Q2. What are the causes of pathologic halitosis?
Answer

1. Periodontal infection: Odor from subgingival dental biofilm. Specific diseases like acute necrotizing ulcerative gingivitis and pericoronitis.
2. Tongue coating harbors microorganisms.
3. Stomatitis, xerostomia.
4. Faulty restorations retaining food and bacteria.
5. Unclean dentures.
6. Oral pathologic lesions like oral cancers, candidiasis.
7. Parotitis, cleft palate.
8. Aphthous ulcers, dental abscesses.

Q3. What are the extraoral factors for halitosis?
Answer

1. Nasal infections like rhinitis, sinusitis, tumors and foreign bodies.
2. Diseases of gastrointestinal tract (GIT) like hiatus hernia, carcinomas, gastroesophageal reflux disorder (GERD).
3. Pulmonary infections like bronchitis, pneumonia, tuberculosis and carcinomas.
4. Certain hormonal changes that occur during ovulation, menstruation, pregnancy and menopause.
5. Systemic diseases like diabetes mellitus, hepatic failure, renal failure, uremia, blood dyscrasias, rheumatologic diseases, dehydration and fever, cirrhosis of liver.

Q4. What are the different tests for detection of halitosis?
Answer

The tests used to detect halitosis are as follows:

1. *Subjective organoleptic method:* This has been used as a bench mark for oral malodor measurement.
2. *Gas chromatography:* In order to assess oral malodor objectively, a portable industrial monitor has been developed. These machines are specifically designed to digitally measure molecular levels of the three major volatile sulfur compounds (VSCs) in a sample of mouth air (hydrogen sulfide, methyl mercaptan and dimethyl sulfide).
3. *Halimeters:* These machines measure the level of sulfide gas found in a person's breath.
4. *Benzoyl-DL-arginine-naphthylamide (BANA) test:* Some of the bacteria like *Porphyromonas gingivalis*, *Treponema denticola* and *Bacteriodes forsythus* produce waste products that are quite odiferous and as a result contribute in causing bad breath.
5. *Chemiluminescence:* This test involves mixing a sample containing sulfur compound (VSCs) with the mercury compound and the resultant reaction causes fluorescence. This test is highly sensitive.

Q5. What is Diamond probe?
Answer

It is a recently developed instrument, which combines the features of a periodontal probe with detection of volatile sulfur compounds in the periodontal pocket.

It is a modified Michigan 'O' style disposable probe with a silver sulfide sensor.

CHAPTER 15

Pathogenesis of Periodontal Diseases

Q1. What are the important cytokines associated with periodontal diseases?

Answer

1. Interleukin (IL)-1: It upregulates adhesion molecules on endothelial cells, lymphocytes, neutrophils and monocytes. It activates T and B lymphocytes and promotes antibody production.
2. IL-2: It stimulates T cells and enhances clonal expansion of beta cells into plasma cells.
3. IL-4, IL-5 and IL-10: They are produced by TH_2 cells and help in the activation of beta cells into plasma cells and downregulate monocytic response.
4. IL-6.
5. IL-8: It is a strong chemoattractant of polymorphonuclear leukocytes (PMNLs) in low concentrations.
6. Tumor necrosis factor (TNF).
7. Prostaglandin E_2.

Q2. What is endotoxin?

Answer

Endotoxin or lipooligosaccharide (LOS) previously termed as lipopolysaccharide (LPS) is found in the outer membrane of all gram-negative bacteria. They are toxic substances affecting the tissues directly and through activation of the host responses.

Q3. What is the role of bacterial enzymes in periodontal diseases?

Answer

The bacterial enzymes that are capable of contributing to the disease process include collagenases, hyaluronidase, gelatinase, aminopeptidase, phospholipases, and alkaline and acid phosphatases. Destruction of periodontal tissues is by degradation of collagen. *Porphyromonas gingivalis* and some strains of *Aggregatibacter actinomycetemcomitans* have been found to produce collagenase. Bacterial hyaluronidase is capable of altering gingival permeability by allowing the apical proliferation of the junctional epithelium along the root surfaces. Hyaluronidase is found in high concentrations in periodontal pocket.

Q4. What are cytokines?

Answer

Cytokines meaning 'cell protein' is used for molecules, which transmit information or signals from one cell to another. Interleukins, growth factors, chemokines and interferon belong to the family of cytokines.

Q5. Which cells play a central role in immunity and inflammation?

Answer

Mast cells, neutrophils, monocytes/macrophages, T cells, B cells and natural killer cells.

Q6. Classify immune response.

Answer

1. Innate immune response.
2. Adaptive immune response.

Q7. Name the three proinflammatory cytokines.

Answer

Interleukin-1, interleukin-6, tumor necrosis factor.

Q8. Name some anti-inflammatory cytokines.

Answer

Interleukin-4, interleukin-10, interleukin-12, interleukin-13, interleukin-18, interferons, transforming growth factor beta (TGF-β).

Q9. What are gingipains?

Answer

Gingipains are trypsin-like cysteine proteinases produced by *P. gingivalis*.

Q10. What are periodontains?
Answer

Periodontains are cysteine-like enzymes secreted by *P. gingivalis*.

Q11. What is immunity? What are its different types?
Answer

Immunity is described as resistance exhibited by the host against any foreign antigen including microorganisms. Immunity may be innate or acquired.

Innate Immunity
An individual possesses innate immunity since birth because of its genetic and constitutional makeup. It is non-specific in nature.

Acquired Immunity
It is acquired during lifetime and is specific in nature. It is of two types:
1. Active immunity: It could be natural or artificial, which is induced by vaccination.
2. Passive immunity: It could be natural or artificial, which is acquired through antiserum injection.

Q12. Classify immune responses.
Answer

The two types of immune responses are:
1. Humoral or antibody-mediated immunity.
2. Cell-mediated immunity.

Q13. What are cytokines? Name some principal cytokines.
Answer

These are biologically active substances secreted by monocytes, lymphocytes and other cells. They exert a regulatory influence on other cells. Some important cytokines are interleukin-1, IL-2, IL-3, IL-4, IL5, IL-6, TNF-α, interferons, lymphokines, colony stimulating factors.

Q14. What are antibodies?
Answer

Antibodies are substances that are formed in serum and tissue fluids in response to an antigen. It reacts with the antigen specifically and in some observable manner.

Q15. What are antigens?
Answer

An antigen is a substance, which when introduced into a body, evokes immune response to produce a specific antibody with which it reacts in an observable manner.

Q16. What is LPS?
Answer

Lipopolysaccharide (LPS) is a component of cell wall of gram-negative bacteria.

Q17. What are virulence factors? Name some.
Answer

Virulence factors are molecules expressed and secreted by pathogens that enable them to achieve colonization, immunosuppression, immunoevasion, entry into and exit out of cells, obtain nutrition from host.

Virulence factors are very often responsible for causing disease in host because they are often responsible for converting non-pathogenic bacteria into pathogens.

Some of the virulence factors are exotoxins, endotoxins, lipopolysachharides, mycotoxins such as aflatoxin.

Q18. What are prostaglandins?
Answer

Prostaglandins are a group of lipid compounds derived from fatty acids and have important functions in body. They act as mediators and have a variety of physiological effects. Some of their various functions are:
1. Cause constriction/dilation in vascular smooth muscle cells.
2. Sensitize spinal neurons to pain.
3. Cause aggregation/disaggregation of platelets.
4. Induce labor.
5. Decrease intraocular pressure.
6. Regulate inflammatory mediation and calcium movement.
7. Control hormone regulation and cell growth.
8. Act on thermoregulatory center of hypothalamus to produce fever.

Q19. What are toll-like receptors?
Answer

Toll-like receptors are a class of proteins that play a key role in the innate immune system as well as the digestive system. They are single, membrane-spanning, non-catalytic receptors usually expressed in sentinel cells such as macrophages and dendritic cells.

These receptors take part in the activation of cytokines, in phagocytosis, apoptosis and release of interferons. They also form an important link between innate and adaptive immunity through their presence in dendritic cells.

CHAPTER 16

Periodontal Medicine

Q1. How can periodontal infection lead to atherosclerosis?

Answer

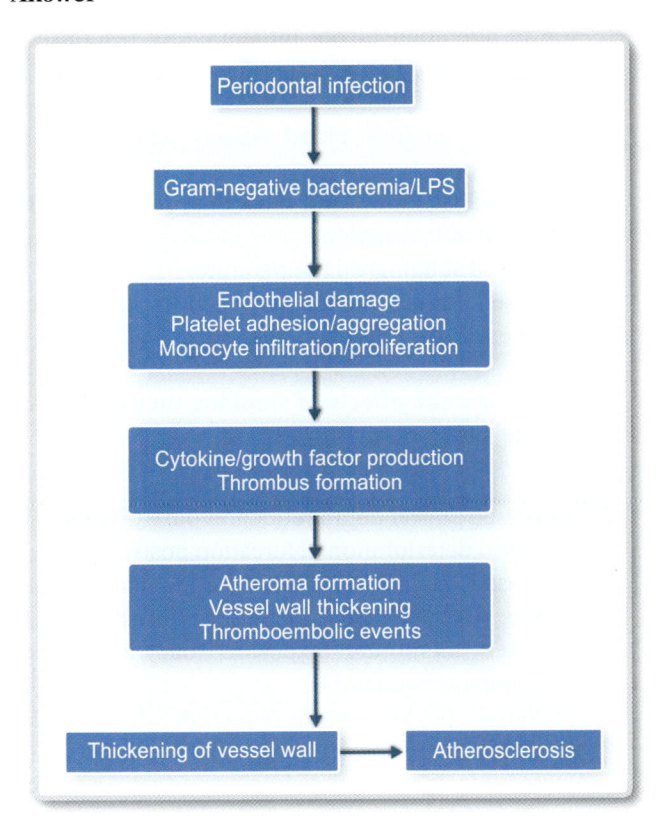

```
Periodontal infection
         ↓
Gram-negative bacteremia/LPS
         ↓
Endothelial damage
Platelet adhesion/aggregation
Monocyte infiltration/proliferation
         ↓
Cytokine/growth factor production
Thrombus formation
         ↓
Atheroma formation
Vessel wall thickening
Thromboembolic events
         ↓
Thickening of vessel wall  →  Atherosclerosis
```

Q2. What is the similarity between chronic obstructive pulmonary disease and periodontal disease?

Answer

Chronic obstructive pulmonary disease shares similar pathogenic mechanism with periodontal disease. In both diseases, a host inflammatory response is mounted in response to chronic challenge by bacteria in periodontal disease and by factors such as cigarette smoking in chronic obstructive pulmonary disease. The resulting neutrophil influx leads to release of oxidative and hydrolytic enzymes that cause tissue destruction directly.

CHAPTER 17

Smoking and Periodontal Disease

Q1. What is the impact of smoking on periodontitis?

Answer

1. Increased prevalence and severity of periodontal destruction.
2. Increased pocket depth, attachment loss and bone loss.
3. Increased rate of periodontal destruction.
4. Increased prevalence of severe periodontitis.
5. Increased tooth loss.
6. Increased prevalence with increased number of cigarettes smoked per day.
7. Decreased prevalence and severity with smoking cessation.

Q2. What is the impact of smoking on gingivitis?

Answer

Decreased gingival inflammation and bleeding on probing.

Q3. What are the effects of smoking on immune system?

Answer

1. Altered neutrophil chemotaxis, phagocytosis and oxidative burst.
2. Increased TNF-α and PGE$_2$ in gingival crevicular fluid (GCF).
3. Increased production of PGE$_2$ by monocyte in response to lipopolysaccharides (LPS).
4. The IgG2 level is reduced suggesting reduced protection against periodontal infection.
5. Nicotine, a major component of tobacco, adversely affects fibroblast function.
6. Nicotine suppresses osteoblast proliferation, while stimulating alkaline phosphatase activity.
7. Tobacco products alter normal reparative and regenerative potential of periodontium.

Q4. What are the effects of smoking on periodontium?

Answer

1. Clinical signs of inflammation are less pronounced, due to alteration in the inflammatory response in smokers or due to alteration in vascular response of gingival tissues.
2. Decreased gingival blood vessels with increased inflammation.
3. Decreased GCF flow and bleeding on probing with increased inflammation.
4. Decreased subgingival temperature.
5. Increased time needed to recover from local anesthesia.

Q5. What are the effects of smoking on periodontal surgeries?

Answer

1. Decreased pocket depth reduction postsurgery.
2. Increased deterioration of furcation postsurgery.
3. Decreased gain in clinical attachment level, decreased bone fill, increased recession and increased membrane exposure following guided tissue regeneration (GTR).
4. Decreased pocket depth reduction after DFDBA allograft.
5. Decreased pocket depth reduction and gain in clinical attachment level after open flap debridement.

Q6. What are the effects of smoking on non-surgical therapies in periodontics?

Answer

1. Decreased clinical response to scaling and root planing.
2. Decreased reduction in pocket depth.
3. Decreased gain in clinical attachment level.
4. Decreased negative impact of smoking with increased level of plaque control.

CHAPTER 18

Host Modulation in Periodontal Therapy

Q1. What do you understand by host modulation therapy?

Answer

Periodontal disease occurs as a result of host interaction between the plaque biofilm and host responses. Host modulatory therapies (HMT) have been developed or proposed to block the pathways responsible for periodontal tissue breakdown.

Q2. What is the role of host during periodontal diseases?

Answer

Activation of host has both protective and destructive aspects. Protective aspects of host response include recruitment of neutrophils, production of protective antibodies and possibly the release of various anti-inflammatory cytokines including TGF-α, interleukins. On the other hand, perpetuation of the host response due to persistent bacterial onslaught may disrupt the homeostatic mechanism and result in release of mediators including proinflammatory cytokines (e.g. IL-1, IL-6, TNF-α), matrix metalloproteinases (MMPs) and prostaglandin.

Q3. What are matrix metalloproteinases? How do they function?

Answer

The MMPs are a family of zinc and calcium-dependent endopeptidases secreted or released by a variety of infiltrating cells like neutrophils, macrophages and resident cells like fibroblasts, epithelial cells, osteoblasts and osteoclasts found in the periodontium. The major functions of MMPs are to degrade the constituents of the extracellular matrix like laminin, collagen, fibronectin, etc.

CHAPTER 19

Defense Mechanism of Gingiva

Q1. Enumerate the types of defense mechanisms.

Answer

Defense mechanisms can be classified as:
1. Non-specific mechanisms.
2. Mechanisms specific to invading foreign proteins called antigens, which stimulate the immune system.

Q2. What are the methods of collection of gingival crevicular fluid (GCF)?

Answer

Gingival crevicular fluid is usually collected from the anterior teeth (least contamination).
 A few techniques are available:
1. Absorbing paper strips (intrasulcular or extrasulcular).
2. Sampling by means of micropipettes.
3. Gingival washings.
4. Other methods (plastic strips and platinum loops).

Q3. Name the stain used for measuring the volume of GCF.

Answer

Ninhydrin stain—gives blue or purple color.

Q4. Name the electronic device used for quantitative estimation of GCF.

Answer

Periotron.

Q5. Name the different models of periotron.

Answer

- Periotron 600
- Periotron 6000
- Periotron 8000.

Q6. What are the drugs that have been detected in GCF?

Answer

Tetracycline and other drugs like minocycline, erythromycin, clindamycin and metronidazole.

Q7. Name the predominant immunoglobulin present in GCF and saliva.

Answer

- In GCF: IgG
- In saliva: IgA.

Q8. Define orogranulocytes.

Answer

In normal individuals, 30,000 neutrophils per minute enter the oral cavity via gingival sulcus across the junctional epithelium. This flow of neutrophils is important to maintain normal periodontal health. These viable neutrophils present in the saliva are known as orogranulocytes. The oral leukocyte migratory rate index (OMRI) allows an objective assessment of periodontal health.

Q9. What are the various conditions in which GCF production is increased?

Answer

1. During inflammation.
2. By mechanical stimulation, e.g. toothbrushing, mastication.
3. Smoking, pregnancy and use of hormonal contraceptives.
4. Transient increase after periodontal surgery.

Q10. What are the contents of GCF?

Answer

1. Cellular elements:
   a. Epithelial cells.
   b. Leukocytes.
   c. Bacteria.
2. Electrolytes:
   a. Sodium.
   b. Potassium.
   c. Calcium.
3. Organic compounds:
   a. Carbohydrates.
   b. Proteins:
      - Immunoglobulins
      - Complement components.
   c. Lipids.
4. Metabolic and bacterial products:
   a. Lactic acid.
   b. Hydroxyproline.
   c. Prostaglandins.
   d. Urea.
   e. Endotoxins.
   f. Cytotoxic substances.
   g. Antibacterial factors.
5. Enzyme and enzyme inhibitors:
   a. Acid phosphatase.
   b. Alkaline phosphatase.
   c. Pyrophosphatase.
   d. Beta-glucuronidase.
   e. Lysozyme.
   f. Hyaluronidase.
   g. Proteolytic enzymes:
      - Mammalian proteinases
      - Bacterial proteinases
      - Serum proteinase inhibitors.
   h. Lactic dehydrogenase.

Q11. What is the clinical significance of GCF?

Answer

General Health and Gingival Fluid

1. Gingival fluid flow and sex hormones: Three groups of females are studied:
   a. First group (during menstruation): There is increase in the gingival fluid flow because the sex hormones (estrogen and progesterone) cause increase in the gingival vascular permeability.
   b. Second group (females on birth control pills): There is significant increase in the amount of exudate recorded.
   c. Third group (females during pregnancy): The gingival exudates reached maximum values during the last trimester and decreased to minimum after delivery.
2. Gingival fluid in diabetic patients: The gingiva of diabetic patients significantly showed higher incidence of vascular modifications, which could be an increase in the width of the basal membrane of capillaries, small arteries and venules, resulting in higher production of gingival fluid. The exudates collected from the diabetic patients showed significantly more levels of glucose than that collected from healthy individuals.

Drugs in Gingival Fluid

Drugs that have been detected in human gingival crevicular fluid (GCF) are tetracycline, minocycline, erythromycin, clindamycin and metronidazole.

Influence of Mechanical Stimuli

Mechanical stimulation of the marginal gingiva, such as massage by means of a round instrument, causes a significant increase in the permeability of the blood vessels located below the junctional and sulcular epithelia.

Smoking: It produces an immediate, but transient increase in GCF flow.

Periodontal Therapy and Gingival Fluid

Measurements of gingival fluid flow have been performed before and after different types of periodontal therapy:
1. Oral prophylaxis: It causes a decrease in the fluid flow, 1 week after oral prophylaxis and then slowly returned to pretreatment values.
2. After surgical procedure: After 1 week of gingivectomy, there was a striking increase in the gingival fluid flow due to the increased inflammatory cells in the smear from the sulci.

Q12. What are the functions of saliva?

Answer

Functions of saliva		
Functions	Salivary components	Probable mechanism
Lubrication	Glycoproteins, mucoids	Coating similar to gastric mucin
Physical protection	Glycoproteins, mucoids	Coating similar to gastric mucin
Cleansing	Physical flow	Clearance of debris and bacteria
Buffering	Bicarbonate and phosphate	Antacids
Tooth integrity maintenance	Minerals, glycoprotein pellicle	Maturation, remineralization, mechanical protection
Antibacterial action	IgA Lysozyme Lactoperoxidase	Control of bacterial colonization Breaks bacterial cell walls Oxidation of susceptible bacteria

CHAPTER 20

Gingival Inflammation

Q1. Define gingivitis.

Answer

The American Academy of Periodontology (AAP) defines gingivitis as an inflammation confined to the tissues of the marginal gingiva.

Q2. Define pristine gingiva.

Answer

Pristine gingiva is a state of super health, where normal gingiva is free from significant accumulation of inflammatory cells. Hence, histologically it may be described as pristine gingiva.

Q3. What are the different stages of gingival inflammation?

Answer

1. Stage I gingivitis: The initial lesion.
2. Stage II gingivitis: The early lesion.
3. Stage III gingivitis: The established lesion.
4. Stage IV gingivitis: The advanced lesion.

Q4. What is subclinical gingivitis?

Answer

In stage I gingivitis, clinically, no visible changes are seen except the presence of exudation of fluid from the gingival sulcus, hence this condition is called subclinical gingivitis.

Q5. What are the time frames of prominent immune cells in different stages of gingivitis?

Answer

Stages of gingivitis	Time period	Immune cell
Stage I	2–4 days	Polymorphonuclear leukocytes (PMNs)
Stage II	4–7 days	Lymphocytes (T cells)
Stage III	14–21 days	Plasma cells and B lymphocytes
Stage IV	–	Plasma cells and presence of all inflammatory cells

CHAPTER 21

Clinical Features of Gingivitis

Q1. How do you classify gingivitis?

Answer

1. Depending on course and duration:
   a. Acute gingivitis is of sudden onset and short duration and can be painful.
   b. Subacute is a less severe phase of acute condition.
   c. Recurrent gingivitis either reappears after treatment or disappears spontaneously.
   d. Chronic gingivitis is slow in onset, of long duration, usually painless and the most commonly occurring gingival condition.
2. Depending on distribution:
   a. Localized gingivitis: If the condition is involving a single tooth or group of teeth.
   b. Generalized gingivitis: It involves entire mouth.
   c. Marginal gingivitis: If the inflammation is limited to the marginal gingiva.
   d. Papillary gingivitis: The inflammation is limited to the interdental papilla.

When the inflammation spreads to attached gingiva, it is termed as diffuse gingivitis.

Q2. What are the two earliest signs of gingival inflammation?

Answer

1. Increased gingival crevicular fluid production rate.
2. Bleeding on probing from gingival sulcus.

Q3. What are the factors causing gingival bleeding?

Answer

Factors causing gingival bleeding are divided into:
1. Bleeding associated with local factors:
   a. Those factors that result in acute bleeding.
   b. Those factors that cause chronic or recurrent bleeding.
2. Bleeding associated with systemic factors.

Q4. What are the systemic causes of gingival bleeding?

Answer

Systemic factors: It include various systemic diseases:
1. Hemorrhagic diseases including vitamin C deficiency, vitamin K deficiency, platelet disorders such as thrombocytopenic purpura, other coagulation defects such as hemophilia, leukemia and others.
2. Excessive administration of drugs such as salicylates and anticoagulants such as Dicumarol and heparin.

Q5. What are the local causes for the gingival bleeding?

Answer

Acute bleeding: It is caused due to:
1. Toothbrush trauma.
2. Impaction of sharp pieces of hard food.
3. Gingival burns from hot foods or chemicals.
4. In conditions such as acute necrotizing ulcerative gingivitis (ANUG).

Chronic bleeding: The most common causes are:
1. Chronic inflammation due to the presence of plaque and calculus.
2. Mechanical trauma, e.g. from toothbrushing, toothpicks or food impaction.
3. Biting into solid foods such as apples.

Q6. What is the normal color of gingiva?

Answer: Coral pink.

Q7. What are the factors that affect the color of gingiva?

Answer

The factors that affect the color of gingiva are:
1. Tissue vascularity.
2. Degree of keratinization.

3. Thickness of the epithelium.
4. Pigmentation within the epithelium.

Q8. What are the color changes associated with acute and chronic gingivitis?

Answer

Acute gingivitis: Erythematous and bright red due to increased vascularity and decreased keratinization.

Chronic gingivitis: Varying shades of red, reddish blue or deep blue due to vascular proliferation and venous stasis.

Q9. What are the metals that alter the color of gingiva?

Answer: Bismuth, mercury, lead, arsenic and silver.

Q10. What is burtonian line?

Answer

Perivascular precipitation of lead in the subepithelial connective tissue, which leads to deep blue or bluish red linear pigmentation.

Q11. List out the systemic diseases causing color changes.

Answer

1. Addison's disease: Bluish black.
2. Peutz-Jeghers disease: Bluish black.
3. Albright's disease: Bluish black.
4. Jaundice: Yellow.
5. Anemia: Dusky pallor.
6. Leukemia: Cyanotic purplish and blue.

Q12. What is the normal contour of the gingiva?

Answer

Normally, marginal gingiva is scalloped and knife-edged, whereas interdental papilla in the anterior region is pyramidal and posteriorly tent-shaped.

Q13. What are the factors affecting contour of gingiva?

Answer

The factors that maintain normal contour are shape of the teeth and its alignment in the arch, location and size of the proximal contact, and dimensions of facial and lingual gingival embrasures.

Q14. What is normal consistency of gingiva? What are the factors responsible?

Answer

Normal gingiva exhibits a firm and resilient consistency. Factors responsible are cellular and fluid content, and collagenous nature of lamina propria.

Q15. What are the factors responsible for the normal size of gingiva?

Answer

Normal size depends on the sum of the bulk of cellular and intercellular elements and their vascular supply.

Q16. What are the different changes in consistency during disease process?

Answer

Changes in consistency during disease process					
Gingival features	In health	Factors responsible	In disease	Factors responsible	Disease conditions
Consistency	Firm and resilient (except free margins)	Collagenous nature of lamina propria and its contiguity with the mucoperiosteum of alveolar bone; cellular and fluid content of tissue	• Soggy puffiness that pits on pressure • Marked softness and friability • Firm leathery • Diffuse puffiness and softening • Sloughing: Grayish flake-like particle of debris • Vesicle formation	• Chronic gingivitis • Exudative • Fibrotic • Acute gingivitis	• Infiltration by fluids and cells of inflammatory exudates • Degeneration of connective tissue and epithelium • Fibrosis and epithelium proliferation • Diffuse edema of acute inflammatory origin • Necrosis with pseudomembrane formation • Intercellular and intracellular edema

CHAPTER 21 Clinical Features of Gingivitis

Q17. What are the changes associated with size of gingiva?

Answer

In disease, the size is increased, which can be termed as gingival enlargement.

The factors responsible for this are given below.

Non-inflammatory type: Increase in fibers and decrease in cells.

Inflammatory type: Increase in cells and decrease in fibers.

Q18. What is the normal surface texture of gingiva?

Answer

Under normal conditions, gingiva appears to be stippled (orange peel appearance) due to attachment of gingival fibers to the underlying bone.

Q19. What do you mean by stippling?

Answer

Stippling is a form of adaptive specialization or reinforcement for function.

Q20. What are the abnormal changes in surface texture during disease?

Answer

Abnormal changes in surface texture	
Disease	Change
Loss of stippling	Gingivitis (inflammation)
Smooth and shiny	Exudative chronic gingivitis
Firm and nodular	Fibrotic chronic gingivitis
Peeling of surface	Chronic desquamative gingivitis
Leathery texture	Hyperkeratosis
Minutely nodular surface	Non-inflammatory gingival hyperplasia

Q21. What is the cause of stippling?

Answer

Microscopically, alternate rounded protuberance and depressions in the gingival layer may give rise to stippled appearance. The papillary layer of connective tissue projects into these depressions (epithelium).

Q22. What is the normal position of gingiva?

Answer

Normally, the gingiva is attached to the tooth at the cementoenamel junction (CEJ). The normal position of gingiva is 1 mm above the CEJ.

Q23. What are the factors responsible for the normal position of gingiva?

Answer

- Position of teeth in the arch
- Root bone angle
- Mesiodistal curvature of tooth surface.

Q24. What are the changes in position of gingiva during disease process?

Answer

In disease, the position can be shifted either coronally (pseudopocket) or apical to the cementoenamel junction (gingival recession).

Q25. What is gingival recession?

Answer

Gingival recession is defined as the exposure of the root surface by an apical shift in the position of the gingiva.

Q26. What are the types of recession?

Answer

There are two types of recession, i.e. visible, which is clinically observable; and hidden, which is covered by gingiva and can only be measured with probe.

Gingival recession may also be localized or generalized.

Q27. What are actual position and the apparent position?

Answer

Position of the gingiva can be actual or apparent. Actual position is the level of epithelial attachment on the tooth, i.e. from the cementoenamel junction (CEJ) to the probable depth of the pocket, whereas apparent position is the level of crest of the gingival margin, i.e. from the CEJ to the gingival margin.

Q28. What is the classification of recession?

Answer

Two classification systems are available:
1. According to Sullivan and Atkins—shallow-narrow, shallow-wide, deep-narrow and deep-wide.
2. According to PD Miller's—class I, class II, class III and class IV.

Class I: Marginal tissue recession that does not extend to the mucogingival junction. There is no loss of bone or soft tissue in the interdental area.

Class II: Marginal tissue recession that extends to or beyond the mucogingival junction. There is no loss of bone or soft tissue in the interdental area.

Class III: Marginal tissue recession that extends to or beyond the mucogingival junction. In addition, there is loss of bone and/or soft tissue in the interdental area or there is malpositioning of the tooth.

Class IV: Marginal tissue recession that extends to or beyond the mucogingival junction with severe loss of bone and soft tissue interdentally and/or severe malpositioning of the tooth.

Q29. What is the etiology of recession?
Answer

Plaque-induced gingival inflammation is the primary etiological factor responsible for gingival recession; next most common cause is faulty toothbrushing. Other secondary/contributing factors of gingival recession are broadly categorized (for convenience) as:
1. Anatomic factors like tooth malposition, presence of dehiscence and fenestrations, gingival ablation from soft tissues like cheek, lips, etc.
2. Habits like faulty toothbrushing or brushing with hard bristles.
3. Iatrogenic factors: Orthodontic movement in a labial direction and improper restorations.
4. Physiologic factors.

Gingival recession was thought to be a physiologic process related to aging. However, this idea was discarded because there was no convincing evidence for a physiologic shift of the gingival attachment.

Q30. What is the clinical significance of recession?
Answer

1. The exposed root surface may be extremely sensitive.
2. Hyperemia of the pulp may result due to gingival recession.
3. Interproximal recession creates oral hygiene problems thereby resulting in plaque accumulation.
4. Finally, it is esthetically unacceptable.

Q31. What are the changes in gingival contour during disease process?
Answer

In diseased conditions (chronic periodontitis), the marginal gingival may become rounded or rolled, whereas interdental papilla can become blunt and flat.

The various diseased conditions related to gingival contour are:
1. Acute necrotizing ulcerative gingivitis (ANUG): Punched out crater-like depression at the crest of the interdental papilla extending to the marginal gingiva.
2. Desquamative gingivitis: Irregularly shaped denuded areas of gingiva.
3. Gingival recession: Exaggerated scalloping.
4. Stillman's cleft: Apostrophe-shaped indentations extending from and into the gingival margins for varying distances on the facial surface.
5. McCall's festoons: Lifesaver-like enlargement of marginal gingiva (canine and premolar facial region).

CHAPTER 22

Gingival Enlargements

Q1. What is gingival enlargement?

Answer

Current clinical descriptive terminology used to describe increase in size of the gingiva is gingival enlargement and gingival overgrowth.

Q2. Classify gingival enlargement.

Answer

1. According to etiologic factors and pathologic changes, gingival enlargements could be listed out as:
   a. Inflammatory enlargement:
      i. Chronic.
      ii. Acute.
   b. Drug-induced enlargement.
   c. Enlargements associated with systemic diseases:
      i. Conditioned enlargement:
         - Pregnancy
         - Puberty
         - Vitamin C deficiency
         - Plasma cell gingivitis
         - Non-specific conditioned enlargement (granuloma pyogenicum).
      ii. Systemic diseases causing gingival enlargements:
         - Leukemia
         - Granulomatous diseases.
   d. Neoplastic enlargement (gingival tumors):
      i. Benign tumors
      ii. Malignant tumors.
   e. False enlargement.
2. According to location and distribution, gingival enlargement can be classified as follows:
   a. Localized: Gingival enlargement limited to one or more (group of) teeth.
   b. Generalized: Entire mouth, the gingiva is enlarged.
   c. Marginal: Limited to the marginal gingiva.
   d. Papillary: Confined to the interdental papilla.
   e. Diffuse: Involves all the parts of the gingiva, i.e. marginal, attached and interdental gingiva.
   f. Discrete: Isolated sessile or pedunculated tumor-like enlargement.

Q3. What are the different grades of gingival enlargement?

Answer

1. Grade 0: No sign of gingival enlargement.
2. Grade I: Enlargement confined to the interdental papilla.
3. Grade II: Enlargement involves papilla and marginal gingiva.
4. Grade III: Enlargement covers three quarters or more of the crown.

Q4. What are the different types of inflammatory gingival enlargement?

Answer

It can be of two types:
1. Acute inflammatory enlargement, e.g. gingival abscess, periodontal abscess.
2. Chronic inflammatory enlargement, which are again localized/generalized or discrete/tumor-like.

Q5. What are the gingival changes in mouth breathers?

Answer

1. Gingivitis and gingival enlargement are often seen.
2. The gingiva appears to be red and edematous with a diffuse shiny surface at the exposed area.
3. Maxillary anterior region is the common site and their effects are generally attributed to irritation from surface dehydration.

Q6. What is the clinical description and pathogenesis of phenytoin-induced gingival enlargement?

Answer

Clinical Features

1. The overgrowth of the gingiva usually becomes apparent in the first 3 months after phenytoin dosage and is most rapid in the 1st year.
2. Clinically, it starts as a painless, bead-like enlargement of facial and lingual gingival margins and interdental papillae.
3. As the condition progresses, the marginal and papillary enlargement unite and develop into a massive tissue fold covering a considerable portion of the crown, and may interfere with the occlusion.
4. When uncomplicated by inflammation, the lesion is mulberry-shaped, firm, pale-pink and resilient with a minutely lobulated surface and no tendency to bleed.
5. The enlargement characteristically appears to project from beneath the gingival margin from which it is separated by a linear groove.
6. The hyperplasia is usually generalized throughout the mouth, but is more severe in maxillary and mandibular anterior region.
7. It occurs in areas in which teeth are present, but hyperplasia of the mucosa in the edentulous mouth has been reported, but is rare.
8. The presence of the enlargement will result in a secondary inflammatory process that complicates gingival hyperplasia caused by the drug.
9. Secondary inflammatory changes produce red or bluish red discoloration and result in an increased tendency toward bleeding.

Pathogenesis

There are many theories as to why phenytoin causes gingival overgrowth. The most convincing at present is the direct effect of drug or metabolites on the gingival tissue.

Major metabolite of phenytoin is 5-(parahydroxyphenyl) 5-phenylhydantoin (5-p-HPPH).

It is suggested that there are different subpopulation of fibroblasts in gingival tissue, some of which synthesize large amount of protein and collagen (high activity fibroblasts) and others, which are only capable of low protein synthesis (low activity fibroblasts).

'Hassell' suggested that high activity fibroblasts become sensitive to phenytoin, with subsequent increase in collagen production.

Q7. What is the treatment of inflammatory gingival enlargement?

Answer

1. Scaling and curettage: If the size of the enlargement does not interfere with the complete removal of deposits, the enlargement caused due to inflammation is treated by scaling and curettage.
2. Surgical removal: It is indicated for two reasons:
    a. In enlargement with significant fibrotic component that does not undergo shrinkage following scaling and curettage.
    b. If the size of the enlargement interferes with the access to the root surface deposits.
3. Surgical techniques: Include the following:
    a. Gingivectomy technique: The incision should be at least 1–2 mm coronal to the mucogingival line.
    b. Flap operation.

Q8. Name certain drugs that commonly cause gingival enlargement.

Answer

1. Anticonvulsant: Phenytoin.
2. Immunosuppressant: Cyclosporin.
3. Calcium channel blockers: Nifedipine.

Q9. What is the treatment of drug-induced gingival enlargement?

Answer

First Step

1. Oral hygiene reinforcement, chlorhexidine gluconate rinses, scaling and root planing.
2. Possible drug substitution. When it is attempted, it is necessary to allow at least a period of 6–12 months between the discontinuation of the offending drug and the possible resolution of gingival enlargement.
3. Professional recalls.

Second Step

If enlargement persists even after following the above-mentioned approaches, surgical therapy is indicated. There are two surgical options available based on the features it presents:

1. Small areas of enlargement with no attachment loss or bone loss and has good keratinized tissue, gingivectomy is the technique of choice.
2. Large areas of enlargement with presence of osseous defects and limited keratinized gingiva, periodontal flap surgery may be indicated.

Q10. What are the other names of idiopathic gingival fibromatosis?

Answer

Other designated terms include, gingival mitosis, elephantiasis gingivae, diffuse fibroma, idiopathic fibromatosis, hereditary gingival hyperplasia and congenital familial fibromatosis.

Q11. What is the etiology of idiopathic gingival fibromatosis?

Answer

Cause is unknown, hence called idiopathic. Some cases have hereditary basis. But the exact mechanism is not well-understood.

Gingival hyperplasia has been described in 'tuberous sclerosis', which is an inherited condition characterized by a triad of epilepsy, mental deficiency and cutaneous angiofibromas.

Q12. What do you understand by 'combined gingival enlargement'?

Answer

It results when gingival hyperplasia is complicated by secondary inflammatory changes. These changes occur when gingival hyperplasia produces conditions favorable for the accumulation of plaque and interferes with effective oral hygiene measures.

It consists of two components:
1. Primary or basic hyperplasia of connective tissue and epithelium, the origin of which is unrelated to inflammation.
2. Secondary complicating inflammatory component.

Q13. Define and enumerate conditioned gingival enlargement.

Answer

Magnification of an existing inflammation initiated by dental plaque. These groups of diseases include:
1. Some of the hormonal conditions (e.g. pregnancy and puberty).
2. Nutritional diseases such as vitamin C deficiency.
3. Non-specific conditioned enlargement (pyogenic granuloma).

Q14. What are the different types of enlargement in pregnancy?

Answer

There are 2 types:
1. Marginal enlargement.
2. Tumor-like enlargement (pregnancy tumor).

Q15. What are the clinical features of marginal enlargement in pregnancy?

Answer

Clinical Features

1. The enlargement is usually generalized and tends to be more prominent interproximally, than on the facial and lingual surface.
2. The enlarged gingiva is bright red or magenta in color, soft and friable, and has a smooth, shiny surface.
3. Bleeding occurs spontaneously or on slight provocation.

Q16. What is pregnancy tumor?

Answer

It is not a neoplasm, but an inflammatory response to local irritation and is modified by the patient's condition. It usually appears after the first trimester, but may also occur earlier.

Q17. What are the clinical features of pregnancy tumor?

Answer

The lesion appears as a discrete mushroom-like flattened spherical mass that protrude from the interdental papilla or the gingival margin and is attached by a sessile or pedunculated base:
1. It tends to expand laterally and pressure from the tongue and cheek increases its flattened appearance.
2. Color—dusky red or magenta with smooth glistening surface that frequently exhibits numerous deep red, pinpoint markings.
3. Consistency—semifirm, but may have varying degrees of softness and friability.
4. It is usually painless, unless complicated by either accumulation of debris under its margin or interference with occlusion—in which case, painful ulceration may occur.

Q18. What is angiogranuloma?

Answer

Gingival enlargement in pregnancy is also termed as angiogranuloma in order to avoid implication of neoplasm (implicated in terms such as pregnancy tumors or fibrohemangioma).

Q19. What is the treatment of pregnancy-induced gingival enlargement?

Answer

Treatment

1. The aim of the periodontal therapy for pregnant patient is to minimize the potential exaggerated inflammatory response related to hormonal alteration.
2. Meticulous plaque control, scaling and root planing, polishing should be the only non-emergent periodontal procedures performed.
3. The second trimester is the safest time in which treatment may be performed. However, long stressful

appointment and periodontal surgical procedures should be postponed until postpartum.
4. One must be aware of a condition, 'supine hypotensive syndrome' that occurs during the third trimester, which is characterized by a decreased blood pressure, syncope and loss of consciousness. In view of this, the appointments should be kept short and the patient should be allowed to change the position frequently.
5. Fully reclining position should be avoided as far as possible.
6. Medication and radiographs should not be prescribed.
7. In case of marginal and interdental enlargement, scaling and curettage can be performed.
8. In case of a tumor-like enlargement, surgical excision is required, which, if possible, should be postponed until postpartum. During pregnancy, the lesion should be removed surgically, only when it interferes with mastication and causes severe disfigurement, and if the patient willingly wants to get it removed.

Q20. What are the clinical features of pubertal gingival enlargement?

Answer

The enlargement is seen in both marginal and interdental papilla, and is characterized by prominent bulbous interproximal papilla. Clinical features include:
1. Frequently, only the facial gingiva is affected.
2. It has all the clinical features associated with chronic inflammatory gingival disease. It is the degree of enlargement and tendency to develop massive recurrence in the presence of relatively little local irritation that distinguishes pubertal gingival enlargement from uncomplicated chronic inflammatory gingival enlargement.
3. Around 11–17 years of age showed a high prevalence of gingival enlargement.
4. The microorganism implicated in pubertal gingival enlargement is *Capnocytophaga*.

Q21. What is the treatment of pubertal gingival enlargement?

Answer

Treatment: It is as follows:
1. Scaling, curettage and oral hygiene instructions.
2. Surgical removal may be performed in severe cases.

Q22. What are the clinical features of vitamin C deficiency?

Answer

Gingival enlargement is marginal and is bluish red, soft, friable and has smooth, shiny surface. Hemorrhage occurring either spontaneously or on slight provocation, and surface necrosis with pseudomembrane formation are common features.

Q23. What is plasma cell gingivitis?

Answer

It is also referred to as atypical and plasma cell gingivostomatitis, and frequently consists of mild-marginal gingival enlargement that extends to attached gingiva. It include the following features:
1. Clinically, gingiva appears red, friable and bleeds easily. An associated cheilitis and glossitis have been reported.
2. It is thought to be allergic in origin, possibly related to the components of chewing gum or dentrifices.

Q24. What is non-specific conditioned enlargement?

Answer

It is a tumor-like gingival enlargement that is considered to be an exaggerated conditioned response to minor trauma. The exact nature of the systemic conditioning factor has not yet been identified.

Q25. Name some systemic diseases causing gingival enlargement.

Answer

1. Leukemia.
2. Sarcoidosis.
3. Wegener granulomatosis.

Q26. What is the treatment of leukemic gingival enlargement?

Answer

After the acute symptoms subside, attention is directed to correct the gingival enlargement. The rationale of treatment is to remove the local deposits and to control inflammatory component of the enlargement. It include:
1. Monitor hematological laboratory values daily (bleeding time, clotting time, partial thromboplastin time and platelet count).
2. Administer antibiotics prior to any periodontal therapy.
3. Extract all hopeless, non-maintainable or potentially infectious teeth, at least 10 days prior to initiation of chemotherapy.
4. Thorough periodontal debridement (scaling and root planing) is done and oral hygiene instructions are given.
5. If there is an irregular bleeding time, careful debridement with cotton pellets soaked in hydrogen

peroxide may be performed around the neck of the teeth.
6. During acute phases of leukemia, patients should receive only emergency periodontal care.

Q27. What are the instructions, which should be followed in leukemic gingival enlargement patients?

Answer

In leukemic patients, the following instructions should be followed (in general):
1. Refer the patient to the physician for medical evaluation and treatment. For this, close cooperation with the physician is required.
2. Prior to chemotherapy, a complete periodontal treatment plan should be prepared with the physician, because once the chemotherapy is started, the patient will become immunosuppressed, thus increasing the risk of secondary infection.

Q28. What is the treatment of acute gingival or periodontal abscess?

Answer

Treatment: It is as follows:
1. Systemic antibiotics.
2. Gentle incision and drainage.
3. Cleanse the area with cotton pellets saturated with 3% hydrogen peroxide.
4. Apply topical pressure with gauze for 15–20 minutes.

Q29. Name some benign tumors of gingiva.

Answer

- Fibroma
- Papilloma
- Peripheral giant cell granuloma
- Central giant cell granuloma
- Leukoplakia
- Gingival cyst.

Q30. Name some malignant tumors of oral cavity causing gingival enlargement.

Answer

- Carcinoma
- Malignant melanoma
- Sarcoma, most commonly Kaposi's sarcoma
- Metastasis.

Q31. What is false enlargement?

Answer

These are not true enlargements of gingival tissues, but may appear as a result of increase in size of the underlying osseous or dental tissues.

Q32. What are the osseous defects that cause gingival enlargement?

Answer

Osseous defects most commonly in tori and exostosis, but it can also occur in Paget's disease, fibrous dysplasia, cherubism, central giant cell granuloma, osteoma and osteosarcoma.

Q33. What are the underlying dental defects that cause false enlargement? What is developmental enlargement?

Answer

During the various stages of eruption of primary dentition, the gingiva may show bulbous, marginal distortion caused by the superimposition of the bulk of the gingiva on the normal prominence of the enamel in the gingival half of the crown. This enlargement has been termed as developmental enlargement.

CHAPTER 23

Acute Gingival Infections

Q1. What is necrotizing ulcerative gingivitis (NUG)?

Answer

Necrotizing ulcerative gingivitis (NUG) is an inflammatory, destructive disease of the gingiva, which presents characteristic signs and symptoms. It can occur in acute, subacute and recurrent forms.

Q2. What are the other names of NUG?

Answer

Other terms used to describe this condition are:
- Vincent's infection
- Trench mouth
- Acute ulceromembranous gingivitis and others.

Q3. What is necrotizing ulcerative gingivitis (NUG)?

Answer

Necrotizing ulcerative gingivitis can cause destruction of the supporting structures. When it involves the bone, it causes bone loss, the condition is referred as necrotizing ulcerative periodontitis.

Q4. What are the oral signs and symptoms of NUG?

Answer

Oral Signs

1. Lesions are characterized by punched out, crater-like depressions at the crest of the interdental papillae, subsequently involving marginal gingiva and rarely attached gingiva.
2. These craters are covered by grayish pseudomembranous slough, which is demarcated from the remaining of the mucosa by a pronounced linear erythema.
3. The ulcerations of NUG could be of two types—lateral ulceration and necrosis, deep ulceration and necrosis.
4. Other signs include gingival hemorrhage or pronounced bleeding on the slightest stimulation.
5. Fetid odor and increased salivation.

Oral Symptoms

1. The lesions are extremely sensitive to touch.
2. The patient complaints of a constant radiating, gnawing pain that is intensified by eating spicy or hot foods and chewing.
3. There is a metallic foul taste and the patient is conscious of an excessive amount of 'pasty saliva'.

Q5. What are the local and systemic predisposing factors for ANUG?

Answer

Local Predisposing Factors

Most important predisposing factors are:
1. Pre-existing gingivitis.
2. Injury to the gingiva.
3. Smoking.

Systemic Predisposing Factors

1. Nutritional deficiency.
2. Debilitating diseases.
3. Psychosomatic factors like stress.

Q6. Which are the microorganisms commonly implicated in ANUG?

Answer

Loesche and colleagues described a constant and a variable flora associated with ANUG.

Q7. What are the different stages of acute necrotizing ulcerative gingivitis (ANUG)?

Answer: According to Horning and Cohen.

Stages	Involvement of the lesion	Cases (%)	Clinical conditions
1	Necrosis of the tip of the interdental papilla	93	Necrotizing ulcerative gingivitis (NUG)
2	Necrosis of the entire papilla	19	Necrotizing ulcerative gingivitis (NUG) or necrotizing ulcerative periodontitis (NUP)
3	Necrosis extending to the gingival margin	21	Necrotizing ulcerative periodontitis
4	Necrosis extending also to the attached gingiva	1	Necrotizing ulcerative periodontitis
5	Necrosis extending into buccal or labial mucosa	6	Necrotizing stomatitis
6	Necrosis exposing alveolar bone	1	Necrotizing stomatitis
7	Necrosis perforating skin of cheek	0	Noma

Q8. What is the role of bacteria in ANUG?

Answer

The specific cause of necrotizing ulcerative gingivitis has not been established. The common opinion is that it is produced by a complex of bacterial organisms, but requires underlying tissue changes to facilitate the pathogenic activity of the bacteria.

Constant flora is composed of fusospirochetal organisms and also *Bacteroides intermedius*. The variable flora consists of a heterogeneous array of bacterial types. These bacteriologic findings have been supported by immunologic data, increased IgG and IgM antibody titers to spirochetes (intermediate sized up to 90%) and *Prevotella intermedia* has been demonstrated. Electron microscopic studies have demonstrated three types of spirochetes, small, intermediate sized (maximum number up to 90%) and large spirochetes.

Q9. What are the four zones described by Listgarten in histopathology of ANUG?

Answer

1. *Zone I—Bacterial zone:* It is the most superficial zone, consists of varied bacteria, including a few spirochetes of the small, medium-sized and large types.
2. *Zone II—Neutrophil-rich zone:* Contains numerous leukocytes predominantly neutrophils with bacteria including spirochetes of various types.
3. *Zone III—Necrotic zone:* Consists of a dead tissue cells, remnants of connective tissue fragments and numerous spirochetes.
4. *Zone IV—Zone of spirochetal infiltration:* Consists of a well-preserved tissue infiltrated with spirochetes of intermediate and large-sized without other organisms.

Q10. What is the differential diagnosis of ANUG?

Answer

Differential diagnosis includes:
- Gonococcal stomatitis
- Agranulocytosis
- Vincent's angina
- Desquamative gingivitis
- Necrotizing ulcerative gingivitis in leukemia
- Necrotizing ulcerative gingivitis in AIDS
- Streptococcal gingivostomatitis.

Q11. What type of mouthwash is commonly preferred in ANUG?

Answer

Rinse the mouth every 2 hours with a diluted 3% hydrogen peroxide (H_2O_2).

Q12. What is the sequence of treatment for ANUG?

Answer

Treatment

1. *Non-ambulatory patient:* With symptoms of generalized systemic complications.
2. *Ambulatory patient:* With no serious systemic complications.

Treatment for Non-ambulatory Patients

Day 1

1. Local treatment limited to gently removing the necrotic pseudomembrane with a pellet of cotton saturated with hydrogen peroxide (H_2O_2).
2. Advised bedrest and rinse the mouth every 2 hours with a diluted 3% H_2O_2.
3. Systemic antibiotics like penicillin or metronidazole can be prescribed.

Day 2

If condition is improved, proceed to the treatment described for ambulatory patients. If there is no improvement at the end of the 24 hours, a bedside visit should be made. The treatment again includes gently swab the area with H_2O_2, instructions of the previous day are repeated.

Day 3

In most cases, the condition will be improved; start the treatment for ambulatory patients.

Treatment for Ambulatory Patients

First visit: A topical anesthetic is applied and after 2 or 3 minutes, the areas are gently swabbed with a cotton pellet to remove pseudomembrane and non-attached surface debris. After the area is cleansed with warm water, the superficial calculus is removed with ultrasonic scalers. Patients with moderate or severe necrotizing ulcerative gingivitis and local lymphadenopathy, are placed on antibiotic regime of amoxicillin 500 mg thrice daily, for penicillin-sensitive patients azithromycin 500 mg once a day for three days or metronidazole 200 mg or 400 mg twice daily for 7 days. Subgingival scaling and curettage are contraindicated at this time because of possibility of extending the infection to deeper tissues.

Instructions to the patient:
1. Avoid smoking and alcohol.
2. Rinse with 3% H_2O_2 and warm water for every 2 hours.
3. Confine toothbrushing to the removal of surface debris with a bland dentifrice, use of interdental aids and chlorhexidine mouthrinse are recommended.

Second visit: Scalers and curettes are added to the instrumentarium. Shrinkage of the gingiva may expose previously covered calculus, which is gently removed. Same instructions are reinforced.

Third visit: Scaling and root planing are repeated, plaque control instructions are given. Hydrogen peroxide rinses are discontinued.

Fourth visit: Oral hygiene instructions are reinforced and thorough scaling and root planing are performed.

Fifth visit: Appointments are fixed for treatment of chronic gingivitis, periodontal pockets and pericoronal flaps and for the elimination of all local irritants. Patient is placed on maintenance program.

Q13. What is acute herpetic gingivostomatitis (AHG)?

Answer

It is a viral infection of the oral mucous membrane caused by herpes simplex virus-I and -II (HSV-I and -II). It occurs most frequently in infants and children younger than 6 years of age, but is also seen in adults.

Q14. What are the oral signs and symptoms of AHG?

Answer

Oral Signs

1. It appears as a diffuse, shiny erythematous, involvement of the gingiva and the adjacent oral mucosa with varying degrees of edema and gingival bleeding.
2. In its initial stage, it may appear as discrete, spherical clusters of vesicles dispersed in different areas, e.g. labial and buccal mucosa, hard palate, pharynx and tongue. After approximately 24 hours, the vesicles rupture and form painful shallow ulcers with scalloped borders and surrounding erythema.
3. Diffuse, edematous, erythematous enlargement of the gingiva with a tendency toward bleeding is seen.
4. The course of the disease is 7–10 days.

Oral Symptoms

1. Generalized soreness of the oral cavity, which interferes with eating and drinking.
2. The ruptured vesicles are sensitive to touch, thermal changes and food.

Q15. What is the etiology for AHG?

Answer

Acute herpetic gingivostomatitis is caused by herpes simplex virus with a size of approximately 100–200 μm.

Q16. Name some herpes virus that cause orofacial diseases in humans.

Answer

Herpes viruses that cause orofacial diseases in humans are:
1. *Herpes virus type 1 (infections above the waist):* Oropharyngeal lesions responsible for acute herpetic gingivostomatitis (HGS) and cold sores.
2. *Herpes virus type 2 (infections below the waist):* Also affects the mouth with changing sexual practices.
3. *Cytomegalovirus:* Severe oral ulcerations.
4. *Varicella zoster virus:* Responsible for chickenpox and herpes zoster (shingles).
5. *Epstein-Barr virus:* Responsible for infectious mononucleosis and hairy leukoplakia.
6. *Human herpes virus 8:* Kaposi's sarcoma.

Q17. What are Lipschutz bodies?

Answer

The vesicle formation in AHG results from fragmentation of the degenerated epithelial cells. Occasionally, round eosinophilic inclusion bodies are found in the nuclei of epithelial cells. These inclusion bodies may be a colony of virus particles, degenerated protoplasmic remnants of the affected cell, or a combination of both, called Lipschutz bodies.

Q18. How the diagnosis of AHS is made?
Answer

Diagnosis is usually established from the patients' history and the clinical findings. For confirmatory tests, the material may be obtained from the lesion and submitted to the laboratory:
1. Herpes simplex virus (HSV) isolation by cell culture is the gold standard.
2. Polymerase chain reaction from swabs obtained by scraping oral lesions.
3. *Tzanck smear:* The material is obtained from the base of the lesion and smeared and stained. The finding of multinucleated cells with swelling, ballooning and degeneration is adequate for diagnosis.

Q19. Which is the stain used in AHG histopathology?
Answer

Smear obtained is Tzancks smear and the stain used is Giemsa's stain.

Q20. What is the differential diagnosis of AHG?
Answer

1. Necrotizing ulcerative gingivitis.
2. Erythema multiforme.
3. Stevens-Johnson syndrome.
4. Aphthous stomatitis (canker sores).

Q21. What is the sequence for treatment of AHG?
Answer

Primary gingivostomatitis is treated with topical lignocaine for pain relief. Acyclovir at 15 mg/kg five times a day for 5–7 days reduces the duration of fever, halts the progression of lesions and reduces infectivity.

Herpes labialis can be managed with topical antiviral medications such as 5% acyclovir cream or 3% penciclovir cream applied three to five times a day at the first sign of the lesion.

Q22. What is recurrent aphthous stomatitis (RAS)?
Answer

Recurrent aphthous stomatitis (aphthae/canker sores) is a common condition, which is characterized by multiple recurrent, small, round or ovoid ulcers with circumscribed margins, erythematous halo and yellow or gray floors typically presenting first in childhood or adolescence.

Q23. What are the different forms of aphthous stomatitis?
Answer

Aphthous stomatitis may occur in the following forms:
1. *Minor aphthae:* It is the most common form, affecting about 80% of patients with RAS. Ulcers are round or oval, usually less than 5 mm in diameter with a gray-white pseudomembrane and an erythematous halo. The ulcers heal within 10–14 days without scarring.
2. *Major aphthae:* It is a rare severe form of aphthous ulcer. Ulcers are oval and may exceed 1 cm in diameter. Ulcers persist for up to 6 weeks and often heal with scarring.
3. *Herpetiform aphthae:* It is the least common variety and is characterized by multiple recurrent crops of widespread small, painful ulcers. As many as 100 ulcers may be present at a given time, each measuring 2–3 mm in diameter.

Q24. Explain the etiology for RAS.
Answer

Etiology is unknown. Major factors linked to RAS are genetic predisposition, hematinic deficiencies, immunologic abnormalities, stress, food allergy and gastrointestinal disorders. Predisposing factors include hormonal disturbances, trauma, cessation of smoking and menstruation.

Q25. How to distinguish between ANUG and AHS?
Answer

Distinction between necrotizing ulcerative gingivitis and primary herpetic gingivostomatitis	
Necrotizing ulcerative gingivitis (NUG)	*Primary herpetic gingivostomatitis (PHG)*
Etiology: Host bacterial interaction, mostly fusospirochetes	Specific viral etiology
Necrotizing condition	Diffuse erythema and vesicular eruptions
Punched out crater-like lesions affecting marginal gingiva; the lesions are covered with pseudomembranous slough, other oral tissues are rarely affected	Vesicles rupture leaving slightly depressed oval and spherical ulcer, diffuse involvement of gingiva, may include buccal mucosa and lips
Uncommon in children	Occurs more frequently in children
No definite duration	Duration of 7–10 days
Not contagious	Contagious

CHAPTER 24

Periodontal Diseases in Children and Young Adolescents

Q1. What are the anatomic considerations or changes of periodontium in children?

Answer

Changes in Gingiva

1. The gingival tissues are more reddish due to a thinner epithelium, a lesser degree of cornification and a greater vascularity.
2. The gingiva lacks the stippling due to shorter and flatter papillae from the lamina propria. Normally, stippling appears at about 3 years of age and occurs in 35% of children between the age of 5 and 15 years.
3. The gingival margins appear to be rounded or rolled due to hyperemia and edema that follows eruption.
4. Greater sulcular depth, due to relative ease of gingival retraction.
5. The gingiva appears to be flabbier due to the lower density of the connective tissue in the lamina propria.

Cementum

1. The cementum is thinner and less dense, and shows a tendency to hyperplasia of cementum apical to the epithelial attachments.

Periodontal Ligament

1. The periodontal ligament in children is wider, has fewer and less dense fibers per unit area. It also has increased hydration with a greater blood and lymph supplies than in adults.

Alveolar Bone

1. In children, the lamina dura is thinner, have fewer trabeculae and larger marrow spaces. There is also a smaller amount of calcification, greater blood and lymph supply and the crest of the alveolar bone appears flatter.
2. The contact points between the deciduous teeth are not as tight as those between the permanent dentition.

Q2. Why the progression of gingivitis to periodontitis is very rare in children?

Answer

The inflammatory response in a child to chronic gingivitis is dominated by T lymphocytes and in adults it is B lymphocytes, this difference might explain why the disease progression from gingivitis to periodontitis is rare.

Q3. Name the predominant microorganisms found in children's plaque.

Answer

Species (in greater number) in children's plaque	Species in adult plaques
• Leptotrichia	• Fusobacterium
• Capnocytophaga	• Eubacterium
• Selenomonas	
• Bacteroides	

Q4. Classify periodontal disease in children.

Answer

Gingival Lesions

1. Acute gingivitis:
   - Herpetic gingivostomatitis
   - Necrotizing ulcerative gingivitis
   - Candidiasis.
2. Chronic marginal gingivitis:
   - Plaque induced
   - Puberty gingivitis.
3. Factitious gingivitis.
4. Localized gingival recession.

Periodontal Lesions

Early Onset Periodontitis
- Prepubertal:
  – Localized
  – Generalized.

- Juvenile:
  - Localized
  - Generalized.

Periodontitis Associated with Systemic Disease
- Papillon-Lefévre syndrome
- Ehler-Danlos syndrome
- Hypophosphatasia
- Chédiak-Higashi syndrome
- Leukocyte adhesion deficiency
- Neutropenia
- Down syndrome.

Q5. Name the various childhood diseases that can cause alterations in gingiva.

Answer
- Chickenpox (varicella)
- Measles (rubella)
- Scarlet fever
- Diphtheria.

CHAPTER 25

Desquamative Gingivitis

Q1. What is desquamative gingivitis?

Answer

Chronic desquamative gingivitis was coined by Prinz in 1932 to describe a peculiar condition characterized by intense erythema, desquamation and ulceration of the free and attached gingiva.

Q2. Classify various desquamative conditions/What are the various gingival conditions that resemble desquamative gingivitis?

Answer

Classification

1. Dermatoses:
   - Oral lichen planus
   - Mucous membrane pemphigoid
   - Pemphigus vulgaris
   - Bullous pemphigoid
   - Erythema multiforme
   - Linear IgA disease
   - Lupus erythematosus
   - Epidermolysis bullosa acquisita
   - Dermatitis herpetiformis.
2. Local hypersensitivity reactions to:
   - Sodium lauryl sulfate
   - Mouthwashes
   - Dental materials
   - Drugs
   - Cosmetics
   - Chewing gum
   - Cinnamon, etc.
3. Miscellaneous:
   - Chronic ulcerative stomatitis
   - Orofacial granulomatosis
   - Plasma cell gingivitis.

Q3. What is Nikolsky's sign?

Answer

A positive Nikolsky's sign is where the surface epithelium 'floats away' when lateral pressure is applied to the mucosa; may indicate vesiculobullous disorders like pemphigus vulgaris.

Q4. What are the clinical features of desquamative gingivitis?

Answer

1. Females are more frequently affected.
2. Buccal aspect of anterior gingiva most commonly affected.
3. The gingiva is fiery red, friable and desquamates easily.
4. Patients complain of soreness, especially when eating spicy or acidic food and of bleeding and discomfort with toothbrushing.
5. Lesions get aggravated by local plaque accumulation.
6. Oral lichen planus, mucous membrane pemphigoid and pemphigus vulgaris are the most commonly associated disorders.
7. A positive Nikolsky's sign.
8. The presence of white plaques or white striae indicates lichen planus.

Q5. Define lichen planus. Describe the types of gingival lesions.

Answer

Lichen planus is an inflammatory mucocutaneous disorder that may involve mucosal surfaces and the skin.

Gingival lesions associated with lichen planus are:
1. Keratotic lesions.
2. Erosive or ulcerative lesions.
3. Vesicular or bullous lesions.
4. Atrophic lesions.

Q6. Which form of lichen planus is most common?
Answer: Reticular form.

Q7. What are civatte bodies?
Answer
These are colloid bodies that are found in histopathological examination of lichen planus.

Q8. Describe histopathological features of lichen planus.
Answer
- Hyperkeratosis
- Basal cell degeneration
- Subepithelial lymphocyte inflammatory infiltrate.

Q9. Where do you see the tombstone appearance of the basal cells?
Answer: Pemphigus vulgaris.

Q10. What are Tzanck cells?
Answer
These are the acantholytic keratinocytes found in histopathological examination of pemphigus vulgaris.

Q11. Describe the treatment for lichen planus and pemphigus.
Answer

Lichen Planus
1. Topical and systemic steroids.
2. Topical tacrolimus or cyclosporine or systemic hydroxychloroquine for unresponsive cases.
3. Surveillance for malignant transformation.

Pemphigus
1. Topical and systemic steroids.
2. The immunosuppressive drugs like azathioprine, cyclophosphamide.
3. Surveillance for relapses.

Q12. What are the characteristic features of erythema multiforme?
Answer

Etiology
Hypersensitivity.

Clinical Features
1. Erosions and ulcerations, which are large and confluent.
2. Severe crusting and bleeding of lips.

Investigations
Histopathology: As follows:
1. Subepithelial or intraepithelial vesiculations.
2. Necrotic keratinocyte.
3. Mixed inflammatory in a perivascular distribution.

Direct immunofluorescence: Fibrin C3 and cytoid bodies at basement membrane zone (BMZ).

CHAPTER 26

Periodontal Pocket

Q1. Define periodontal pocket.
Answer

Pocket can be defined as deepening of the gingival sulcus; if this happens due to coronal migration of the marginal gingiva it is called gingival or pseudopocket. Deepening due to apical migration of the junctional epithelium is referred as 'true pocket'.

Q2. Classify periodontal pockets.
Answer

1. Depending upon its morphology:
   a. Gingival/false/relative pocket.
   b. Periodontal/absolute/true pocket.
   c. Combined pocket.
2. Depending upon its relationship to crestal bone:
   a. Suprabony/supracrestal/supra-alveolar pocket.
   b. Infrabony/intrabony/subcrestal/intra-alveolar pocket.
3. Depending upon the number of surfaces involved:
   a. Simple pocket—involving one tooth surface.
   b. Compound pocket—involving two or more teeth surfaces.
   c. Complex pocket—where the base of the pocket is not in direct communication with the gingival margin. It is also known as spiral pocket.
4. Depending upon the nature of the soft tissue wall of the pocket:
   a. Edematous pocket.
   b. Fibrotic pocket.
5. Depending upon the disease activity:
   a. Active pocket.
   b. Inactive pocket.

Q3. What are the different types of probing depth?
Answer

1. Biologic depth: 1.8 mm.
2. Probing depth: 2–3 mm.

Q4. What are the clinical features of a periodontal pocket?
Answer

Clinical Features
Signs

1. Enlarged, bluish-red marginal gingiva with a 'rolled' edge separated from the tooth surface.
2. A bluish-red vertical zone extending from the gingival margin to the alveolar mucosa.
3. A break in the faciolingual continuity of the interdental gingiva.
4. Shiny, discolored and puffy gingiva associated with exposed root surfaces.
5. Gingival bleeding, purulent exudate from the gingival margin.
6. Mobility, extrusion and migration of teeth.
7. Development of diastema where none had existed previously.

Symptoms

1. Localized pain or a sensation of pressure in the gingiva after eating, which gradually diminishes.
2. A foul taste in localized areas.
3. A tendency to suck material from the interproximal spaces.
4. Radiating pain 'deep in the bone'.
5. A 'gnawing' feeling or feeling of itching in the gums.
6. The urge to dig a pointed instrument into the gums and relief is obtained from the resultant bleeding.
7. Patient complains that 'food sticks between the teeth' or the teeth 'feel loose' or a preference to 'eat on the other side'.
8. Sensitivity to heat and cold; toothache in the absence of caries.

Q5. What is site specificity?

Answer

Periodontal destruction does not occur in all parts of the mouth at the same time, but rather on a few teeth at a time or only some aspect of the tooth. This is referred as site specificity of periodontal disease.

Q6. Explain the pathogenesis of periodontal pocket formation.

Answer

First Event

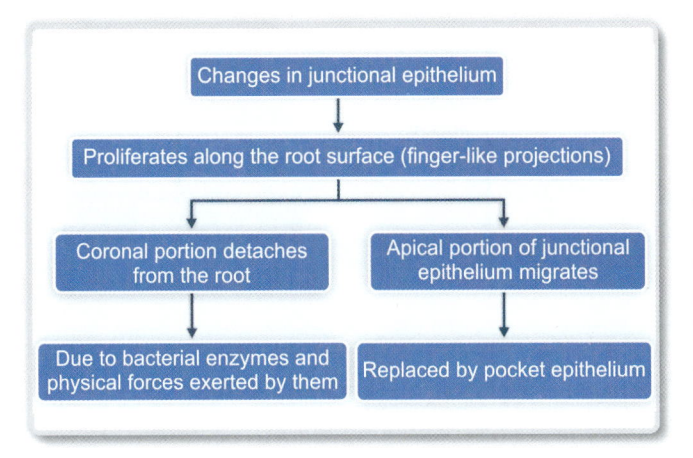

```
Changes in junctional epithelium
            ↓
Proliferates along the root surface (finger-like projections)
            ↓
Coronal portion detaches        Apical portion of junctional
    from the root                   epithelium migrates
            ↓                              ↓
Due to bacterial enzymes and     Replaced by pocket epithelium
physical forces exerted by them
```

Second Event

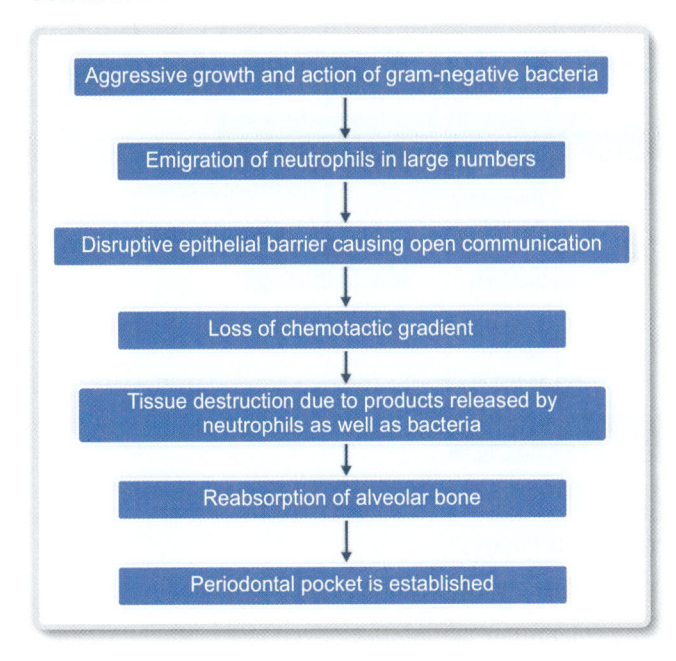

```
Aggressive growth and action of gram-negative bacteria
            ↓
Emigration of neutrophils in large numbers
            ↓
Disruptive epithelial barrier causing open communication
            ↓
Loss of chemotactic gradient
            ↓
Tissue destruction due to products released by
neutrophils as well as bacteria
            ↓
Reabsorption of alveolar bone
            ↓
Periodontal pocket is established
```

Q7. Enumerate the microtopography of periodontal pocket.

Answer

1. Areas of relative quiescence.
2. Areas of bacterial accumulation—mainly cocci, rods, filamentous rods with a few spirochetes.
3. Area of emergence of leukocytes.
4. Areas of leukocyte-bacterial interaction.
5. Areas of intense epithelial desquamation.
6. Areas of ulceration with exposed connective tissue.
7. Areas of hemorrhage with numerous erythrocytes.

Q8. What are the contents of a periodontal pocket?

Answer

It consists of debris, principally containing microorganisms and their products (like enzymes, endotoxins and other metabolic products), dental plaque, gingival fluid, food remnants, salivary mucin, desquamated epithelial cells and leukocytes. If purulent exudate is present, it consists of living, degenerated and necrotic leukocytes (PMNLs), living and dead bacteria, serum and a scanty amount of fibrin. Pus formation is a common feature in periodontal disease, but it is only a secondary sign.

Q9. What are the changes in root surface wall of the pocket?

Answer

Structural Changes

1. Presence of pathologic granules.
2. Areas of increased mineralization.
3. Areas of demineralization/root caries.

Chemical Changes

The mineral content of exposed cementum is increased. The following minerals are increased in diseased root surfaces: calcium, magnesium, phosphate, fluoride and others. Hence, a highly increased, resistant calcified layer to decay is formed. This can also be harmful if the adsorbed products are toxic.

Cytotoxic Changes

Bacterial penetration into the cementum can be found as deep as cementodentinal junction. In addition, bacterial products such as endotoxins have also been detected.

Q10. Enumerate the zones in the base of the pocket.

Answer

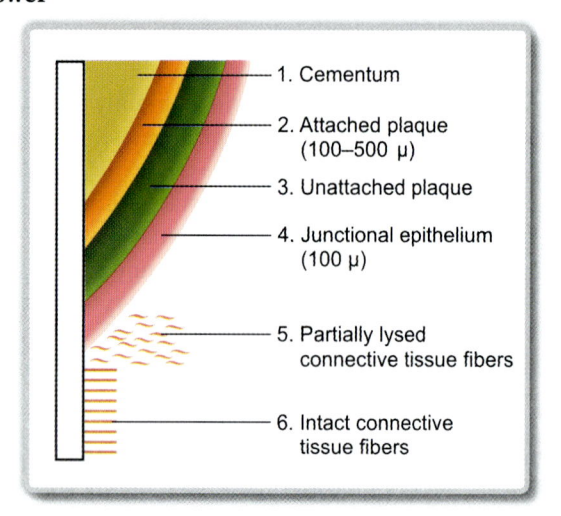

1. Cementum
2. Attached plaque (100–500 μ)
3. Unattached plaque
4. Junctional epithelium (100 μ)
5. Partially lysed connective tissue fibers
6. Intact connective tissue fibers

Q11. What are the methods to determine periodontal pocket?

Answer

- Probing depth measurement
- Clinical detection of attachment loss
- Clinical detection of suprabony and infrabony pockets.

Clinically, probing depth measurement is recorded from the crest of the marginal gingiva to the probable depth of the pocket.

Attachment level is measured from cementoenamel junction to the probable depth of the pocket.

To differentiate between pseudo and true pocket, attachment level measurement should be considered.

Q12. What are the differences between suprabony and infrabony pockets?

Answer

Suprabony pockets	Infrabony pockets
The base of the pocket is coronal to the crest of alveolar bone	The base of the pocket is apical to the crest of the alveolar bone
The pattern of bone destruction is horizontal	The pattern of bone destruction is vertical/angular
Interproximally, the transseptal fibers are arranged horizontally	Interproximally, the transseptal fibers are arranged in an oblique pattern, extending from cementum below the pocket over to the cementum of the adjacent tooth
On the facial and lingual surfaces, the periodontal ligament fibers follow normal horizontal-oblique course between the tooth and bone	On facial and lingual surfaces, the periodontal ligament fibers follow the angular pattern of the adjacent bone

Q13. Explain the treatments of periodontal pocket.

Answer

Treatment of Pockets Depends on the Type of Pocket

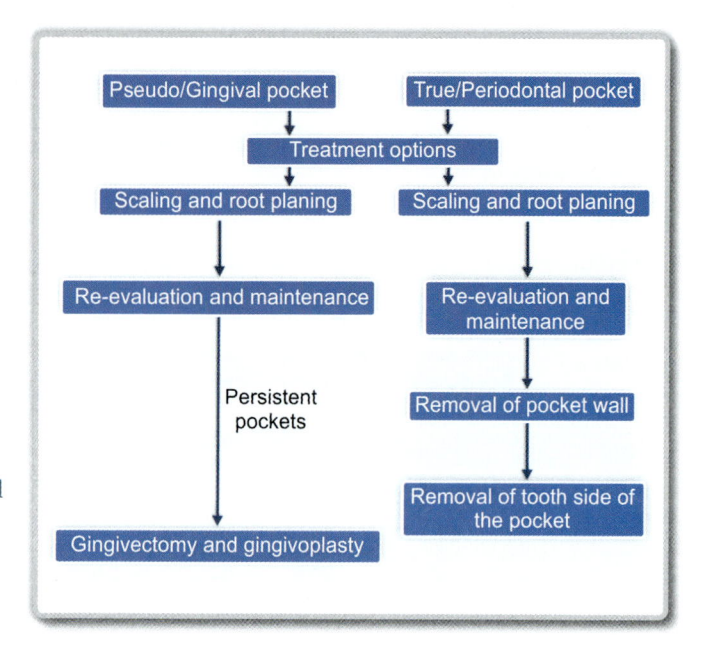

Pseudo/Gingival pocket → Treatment options → Scaling and root planing → Re-evaluation and maintenance → Persistent pockets → Gingivectomy and gingivoplasty

True/Periodontal pocket → Scaling and root planing → Re-evaluation and maintenance → Removal of pocket wall → Removal of tooth side of the pocket

Treatment of Suprabony and Infrabony Pockets

Suprabony → Anterior teeth / Posterior teeth

Anterior teeth → Scaling + root planing and maintenance → Persistent pockets → Curettage → Moderate to severe pockets → Flap surgery utilizing crevicular incisions

Posterior teeth → Scaling + root planing and maintenance → Persistent pockets + inadequate access → Flap surgery

Infrabony → New attachment procedures

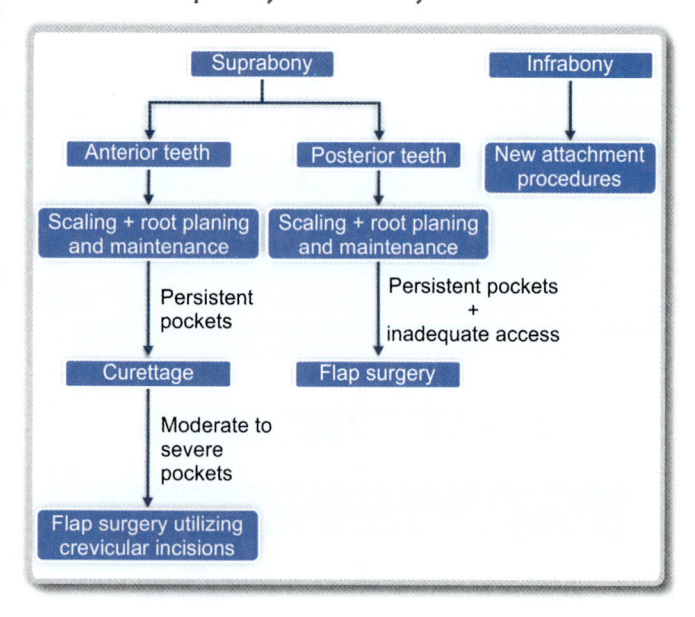

Treatment of Pockets

It can also be classified under three main headings.

New Attachment Techniques

It offers ideal result by reuniting the gingiva to the tooth at a position coronal to the base of pre-existing pocket. Here all the structures of lost periodontium are restored.

Following are the techniques for new attachment:
1. Non-graft associated new attachment procedures.
2. Graft associated new attachment procedures.
3. Combined techniques.

Removal of Pocket Wall

1. Retraction or shrinkage, e.g. scaling and root planing.
2. Surgical removal by gingivectomy or by means of an undisplaced flap.
3. Apical displacement of the pocket wall by apically displaced flap.

Removal of the Tooth Side of the Pocket

By tooth extraction or partial tooth extraction such as hemisection or root resection.

Q14. What are the causes of periodontal abscess?

Answer

Mainly divided into:
1. Abscess related to periodontal diseases.
2. Periodontal abscess caused by other factors (non-periodontitis related abscess).

Periodontal abscess may occur in the following ways:

1. Deep extension of infection from periodontal pocket into the supporting tissues and localization of suppurative inflammatory process along the lateral aspect of the root.
2. Lateral extension of inflammation from inner surface of a pocket into the connective tissue of the pocket.
3. The existence of tortuous pockets, with cul-de-sac that eventually becomes isolated and may favor abscess formation.
4. Incomplete removal of calculus during treatment of a periodontal pocket may lead to occlusion of the pocket orifice due to shrinkage of gingival wall and a periodontal abscess may form in the sealed-off portion of the pocket.
5. Treatment with systemic antibiotics along with root planing in advanced periodontal patients may result in abscess formation.

Other factors that may cause periodontal abscess include:
1. Impactation of foreign bodies especially related to oral hygiene aids (toothbrush bristle, piece of dental floss) have been termed as 'oral hygiene abscess'.
2. Perforation of the lateral wall of root in endodontic therapy.

CHAPTER 27

Bone Loss and Patterns of Bone Destruction

Q1. What are the factors that can lead to bone destruction in periodontal disease?

Answer

Local factors could be:
1. Chronic gingival inflammation.
2. Trauma from occlusion.
3. Combination of both.

Systemic diseases include:
1. Osteoporosis.
2. Hyperparathyroidism.
3. Leukemia.

Q2. What are the effects of trauma from occlusion on bone?

Answer

Trauma from occlusion in the absence of inflammation can cause the following changes:
1. Increased compression and tension of the periodontal ligament.
2. Increased osteoclasis of alveolar bone and necrosis of periodontal ligament.

These changes are reversible, if offending forces are removed. However, persistent trauma from occlusion results in funnel-shaped bony defects.

Q3. What is radius of action?

Answer

On the basis of Waerhaug's measurements, it was postulated that there is a range of effectiveness of about 1.5–2.5 mm within which bacterial plaque can induce bone loss and beyond 2.5 mm, there is no effect. Interproximal angular defects can appear only in spaces wider than 2.5 mm because narrower spaces are destroyed completely. This range of effectiveness is called radius of action.

Q4. How much is the rate of bone loss per year?

Answer

Loe and associates found the rate of bone loss on an average to be about 0.2 mm a year for facial surfaces and about 0.3 mm a year for proximal surfaces, when periodontal disease is allowed to progress untreated.

Q5. Explain the pathway of bone loss.

Answer

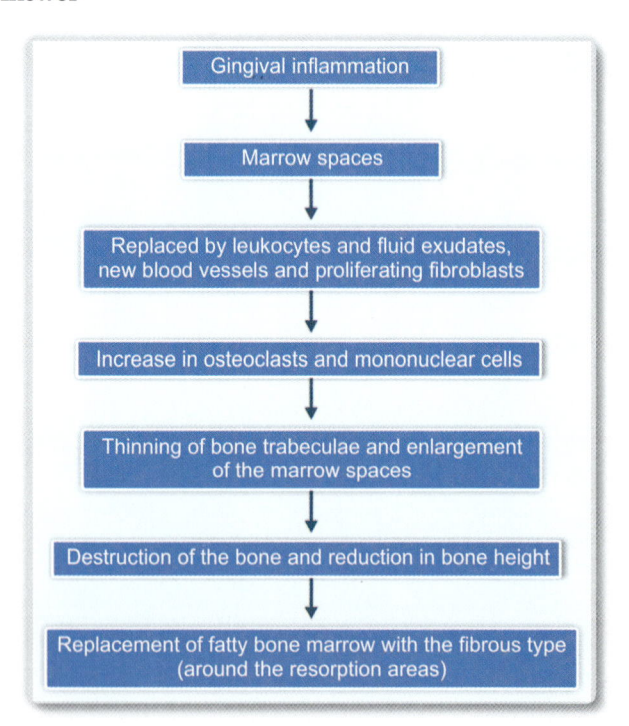

Gingival inflammation
↓
Marrow spaces
↓
Replaced by leukocytes and fluid exudates, new blood vessels and proliferating fibroblasts
↓
Increase in osteoclasts and mononuclear cells
↓
Thinning of bone trabeculae and enlargement of the marrow spaces
↓
Destruction of the bone and reduction in bone height
↓
Replacement of fatty bone marrow with the fibrous type (around the resorption areas)

Q6. What are the different types or patterns of bone destruction in periodontal disease?

Answer

Horizontal Bone Loss

It is the most common pattern of bone loss in periodontal disease. The bone is reduced in height, but the bone margins remain roughly perpendicular to the tooth surface.

Vertical or Angular Defects

They are those that occur in an oblique direction, leaving a hollowed out through in the bone alongside the root. The base of the defect is located apical to the surrounding bone.

Q7. Classify angular defects.

Answer

Angular defects are classified on the basis of number of walls present as:
1. One-walled or the hemiseptal defect—one wall is present.
2. Two-walled defect—two walls are present.
3. Three-walled or intrabony defect—three walls are present (more common on mesial surfaces of upper and lower molars).
4. Combined osseous defect—the number of walls in the apical portion of the defect are greater than that in its occlusal portion. Radiographs may help up to some extent to locate vertical defects, but the best would be surgical exposure of the defect.

Q8. What are osseous craters?

Answer

They are concavities in the crest of the interdental bone confined within the facial and lingual walls. It is found to make up two-thirds of all mandibular defects, can be diagnosed by transgingival probing.

The following reasons have been suggested for the high frequency of interdental craters:
1. Interdental areas are more prone to the accumulation of plaque and are more difficult to clean.
2. The normal flat or even concave faciolingual shape of the interdental septum in lower molars may favor crater formation.
3. Vascular patterns from the gingiva to center of the crest may provide a pathway for inflammation.

Q9. What is reversed architecture?

Answer

These defects are produced by loss of interdental bone, including the facial and lingual plates without concomitant loss of radicular bone, thereby reversing the normal architecture (more common in maxilla).

Q10. What are the different types of bone destruction patterns?

Answer

Bone destruction patterns in periodontal disease are:
1. Horizontal bone loss.
2. Vertical or angular defects.
3. Osseous craters.
4. Bulbous bony contours.
5. Reversed architecture.
6. Edges.
7. Furcation involvement.

Q11. Classify bone defects.

Answer

1. Goldman and Cohen (1958): According to morphology of bone defects, it can be classified as:
   - One-walled defect
   - Two-walled defect
   - Three-walled defect
   - Combined defect.
2. Glickman (1964) classified bony defects as:
   - Osseous/Interdental craters
   - Hemiseptal defects
   - Infrabony defects
   - Ulbous bone contours
   - Inconsistent margins and ledges
   - Reversed architecture.
3. Prichard (1967) expanded the classification and included furcation involvement, anatomic aberrations of the alveolar process, i.e. thick marginal ledges, exostoses and tori, dehiscence and fenestrations.

Q12. What is Glickman's bone factor concept?

Answer

Local and systemic factors regulate the physiologic equilibrium of the bone. The systemic influence on alveolar bone as stated by Glickman considers a systemic component in all cases of periodontal disease and this is known as Glickman's bone factor concept.

CHAPTER 28

Chronic Periodontitis

Q1. Define chronic periodontitis.
Answer

Chronic periodontitis is defined as "an infectious disease resulting in inflammation within the supporting tissues of the teeth, progressive attachment loss and bone loss".

Q2. What are the clinical features of chronic periodontitis?
Answer

Clinical Features
1. Age of onset is usually 30–35 years.
2. The disease is usually generalized, although some areas are more deeply involved than the other areas.
3. No consistent pattern of distribution of lesion is seen, except that they are usually not isolated to one or two sites.
4. Highly acute inflammatory sites are not seen, mostly gingiva appear to be slight to moderately swollen and color may range from pale red to magenta.
5. Loss of stippling, blunt or rolled gingival margins and flattened or cratered papillae may be seen.
6. Spontaneous bleeding and inflammation related exudate from the pockets may also be found.
7. When the pocket occludes, it may result in abscess formation.
8. Pocket depths are variable and both suprabony and infrabony pockets can be found.
9. Conditions that enhance plaque accumulation like the open interdental contacts, defective restorative margins and malposed teeth may be frequently seen.
10. The amount of microbial deposits is consistent with severity of the disease.
11. Tooth mobility is seen in advanced cases.
12. No serum neutrophil or monocyte abnormalities are seen.

Q3. Name the microorganisms that are associated with chronic periodontitis.
Answer

- *Porphyromonas gingivalis (P. gingivalis)*
- *Prevotella intermedia (P. intermedia)*
- *Capnocytophaga*
- *Aggregatibacter actinomycetemcomitans (A. actinomycetemcomitans)*
- *Eikenella corrodens (E. corrodens)*
- *Campylobacter rectus (C. rectus).*

Q4. Differentiate between localized and generalized periodontitis.
Answer

Localized Periodontitis
Periodontitis is considered localized, when less than 30% of the sites assessed in the oral cavity demonstrates attachment loss and bone loss.

Generalized Periodontitis
It is considered generalized, when more than 30% of the sites assessed in the oral cavity demonstrate attachment loss and bone loss.

Q5. What are the different models associated with progression of periodontitis?
Answer

Several models have been proposed to describe the rate of disease progression:
1. Continuous paradigm.
2. Random burst theory.
3. Asynchronous multiple burst hypothesis.

Continuous paradigm implies slow, continuous and progressive destruction of periodontium. This type of progression has been reported in longitudinal studies, not responsive to treatment.

The random burst theory proposes that the progression of disease occurs at short periods of active destruction, which are followed by periods of remission that randomly occur with respect to time and site in an individual.

In asynchronous multiple burst model, the tissue destruction occurs at a definite period of time in one's life and then it passes into a state of remission as in juvenile periodontitis.

Q6. What are the risk factors associated with periodontitis?

Answer

Local Factors

These include plaque and plaque retentive factors:
1. Plaque attached to the tooth and gingival surfaces at the dentogingival junction is considered to be the primary etiologic factor in chronic periodontitis.
2. Plaque retentive factors are those that facilitate plaque accumulation or prevent the removal of plaque by routine oral hygiene procedures. Some of these factors include:
    a. Calculus.
    b. Subgingival and/or overhanging margins of restorations.
    c. Deep carious lesions.
    d. Crowded or malaligned teeth.
    e. Root surface irregularities.

Systemic Factors

The role of systemic factors in periodontal diseases can influence the host response and increase the rate of progression of periodontal disease.
1. Diabetes—mostly type II, a non-insulin dependent diabetes.

Environmental or Behavioral Factors

1. Smoking.
2. Emotional stress.

Genetic Factors

1. Genetic predisposition may be observed in aggressive periodontal breakdown in response to accumulation of plaque and calculus.

CHAPTER 29

Aggressive Periodontitis

Q1. What do you understand by aggressive periodontitis?

Answer

Aggressive periodontitis is characterized by the rapid loss of attachment and bone loss occurring in an otherwise clinically healthy patient with the amount of microbial deposits inconsistent with disease severity and familial aggregation of diseased individuals.

Q2. Define localized aggressive periodontitis and generalized aggressive periodontitis.

Answer

A more recent definition by Genco et al in 1986 describes localized juvenile periodontitis as a disease occurring in otherwise healthy individuals under the age of 30 years with destructive periodontitis localized to the first permanent molars and incisors not involving more than two other teeth.

Generalized juvenile periodontitis is defined as destructive periodontitis in individuals under the age of 30 years affecting more than 14 teeth, i.e. generalized to an arch or an entire dentition.

Q3. What are the striking clinical features of aggressive periodontitis?

Answer

Age and Sex Distribution

Affects both the sexes and is seen mostly between puberty and 20 years of age. Some studies show predilection to female patients.

Distribution of Lesions

Three areas of localization of bone loss have been described:
1. First molar and/or incisors.
2. First molar and/or incisors + additional teeth (not exceeding 14 teeth).
3. Generalized involvement.

For localized juvenile periodontitis, classic distribution is in the first molars and incisors with least destruction in the cuspid, premolar area.

Q4. What are the clinical findings in aggressive periodontitis?

Answer

1. The most striking feature is lack of clinical inflammation despite the presence of deep periodontal pockets.
2. There is a small amount of plaque, which forms a thin film on the tooth and rarely mineralizes to become calculus.
3. Most common initial symptoms are mobility and migration of first molars and incisors. Classically, a distolabial migration of the maxillary incisors with diastema formation occurs, lower incisors rarely migrate compared to upper incisors, all changes followed by sequelae of migration are seen.
4. As the disease progresses, other symptoms like root surface sensitivity, deep dull radiating pain, periodontal abscess formation and regional lymph node enlargement may occur.

Q5. What is the significant radiographic finding in localized aggressive periodontitis (LAP)?

Answer

1. Vertical or angular bone loss around the first molars and incisors in otherwise healthy teenagers is a diagnostic sign of classic juvenile periodontitis. The pattern appears to be "arc-shaped loss of alveolar bone extending from distal surface of second premolar to mesial surface of second molar."
2. Frequently, bilaterally symmetrical patterns of bone loss occur, called 'mirror image pattern'.

Q6. What are different factors involved in pathogenesis of aggressive periodontitis?

Answer

Pathogenesis of aggressive periodontitis is due to interplay of several factors, these include the specific microbiology of subgingival plaque, defects in cementum, hereditary factors, impaired polymorphonuclear neutrophils (PMNs) function and disorders of the immune system.

Q7. What are the microorganisms that are consistently associated with LAP?

Answer

Two types of bacteria are considered to be pathogens in LAP such as *Aggregatibacter actinomycetemcomitans* and *Capnocytophaga*. *A. actinomycetemcomitans* is a short, facultatively anaerobic, non-motile and gram-negative rod.

Q8. Role of immunology in pathogenesis of LAP.

Answer

Immune defects that have been implicated in the pathogenesis of localized aggressive periodontitis are functional defects of polymorphonuclear leukocytes/monocytes, thereby it impairs the chemotactic attraction of polymorphonuclear leukocytes (PMNLs) to the site of infection.

Q9. Clinical characteristics of GAP.

Answer

1. Age and sex distribution: It affects persons between puberty and 35 years (but may be older). No sex discrimination is seen.
2. Distribution of lesion: No specific pattern is observed, all or most of the teeth are affected.
3. Two types of gingival responses may be seen in generalized aggressive periodontitis. One is severe, acutely inflamed tissue that is often proliferating, ulcerated and fiery red, spontaneous bleeding and suppuration are commonly seen. In the other cases, the gingival tissue may appear pink and free of inflammation, but deep pockets can be demonstrated by probing.
4. Some patients may have systemic manifestations such as weight loss, mental depression and general malaise.

Q10. What are various risk factors for aggressive periodontitis?

Answer

1. Microbiologic factors: *A. actinomycetemcomitans* has been implicated as the primary pathogen. Others are *Capnocytophaga sputigena*, *Mycoplasma* subspecies and spirochetes.
2. Immunologic factors: Approximately 75% of patients with LAP have dysfunctional neutrophils, which are seen as decreased in the chemotactic response to several chemotactic agents. Host response is often characterized by defects in either neutrophils or monocytes.
3. Genetic factors: Familial clustering of neutrophil abnormalities may be seen.
4. Environmental factors: Smoking is one of the factors that can influence the extent of destruction seen in young patients.

CHAPTER 30

Necrotizing Ulcerative Periodontitis, Refractory Periodontitis and Periodontitis as a Manifestation of Systemic Disease

Q1. What is NUP?
Answer

Necrotizing ulcerative periodontitis (NUP) occurs as a result of extension of necrotizing ulcerative gingivitis into the periodontal structures, leading to loss of attachment and bone loss.

Q2. What are the two basic types of NUP?
Answer

There are two types of necrotizing ulcerative periodontitis described, based on its relationship to acquired immunodeficiency syndrome (AIDS):
1. Non-AIDS type necrotizing ulcerative periodontitis.
2. AIDS-associated necrotizing ulcerative periodontitis.

Q3. What are the clinical features of non-AIDS type necrotizing ulcerative periodontitis?
Answer

Clinical Features
Since necrotizing ulcerative periodontitis occurs after repeated attacks of necrotizing ulcerative gingivitis (NUG), all the characteristic clinical features of necrotizing ulcerative gingivitis are as follows:
1. Ulceration and necrosis of gingival margin, which gets covered by a pseudomembranous slough.
2. The ulcerated margins are surrounded by an erythematous halo.
3. The lesions are extremely painful and bleed spontaneously.
4. Localized lymphadenopathy, fever and malaise.

These lesions, especially in long-standing cases, can extend to the deeper periodontal structures resulting in deep, crater-like osseous lesions especially in interdental areas. Such cases are identified as necrotizing ulcerative periodontitis. Most striking feature of this condition is absence of deep conventional pockets associated with deep interdental osseous craters.

Q4. What are the clinical features of AIDS-associated necrotizing ulcerative periodontitis?
Answer

Gingival and periodontal lesions of HIV positive patients appear to have similar findings that are seen in non-AIDS-associated necrotizing ulcerative periodontitis patients; in addition, they may exhibit certain complications such as follows:
1. Large areas of soft tissue necrosis with exposure of bone and sequestration of bone.
2. Sometimes these lesions may extend onto the buccal vestibule or the palate and become necrotizing stomatitis.

Q5. Define refractory periodontitis.
Answer

According to American Academy of Periodontology, refractory periodontitis has been defined as "those cases, which do not respond to any treatment provided, whatever the thoroughness or frequency."

Q6. What is the etiology/risk factors responsible for refractory cases?

Answer

1. Abnormal host response.
2. Resistant strains of pathogenic periodontal microflora.
3. Failure to eliminate plaque retentive factors, such as furcation involvement, irregular root surface, palatogingival groove, etc. that may in turn interfere with complete plaque removal.
4. On the other hand, smoking and systemic diseases may result in generalized lesions, which may not respond favorably to treatment.

Specific microorganisms have been identified in lesions of refractory periodontitis. Haffajee et al in 1988 reported three major microbial complexes in refractory periodontitis cases:

1. *Bacteroides forsythus, Fusobacterium nucleatum* and *Campylobacter rectus.*
2. *Staphylococcus intermedius, Porphyromonas gingivalis* and *Peptostreptococcus micros.*
3. *S. intermedius* and *F. nucleatum.*

Q7. Differentiate between refractory and recurrent periodontitis.

Answer

Distinction between recurrent and refractory periodontitis		
Disease	Recurrent periodontitis	Refractory periodontitis
Definition	Sites are successfully treated, but disease returns may refer to site/patients	Sites do not respond to conventional therapy; usually refers to patients, but may refer to sites
Phase of therapy	May be because of inadequate therapy during maintenance/no maintenance	May be because of inadequate therapy during active treatment/other factors
Etiology	May be because of reinfection with microbes that were suppressed, but not eliminated; reinfection with eliminated organisms or new bacteria	May be because of infection with tissue invasive microbes that cannot be eliminated with conventional therapy or because of immunoincompetence
Immune system	Immunocompetent	May not be immunocompetent
Antibiotic therapy	Not usually needed	Usually needed

CHAPTER 31

AIDS and the Periodontium

Q1. Classify periodontal diseases associated with human immunodeficiency virus (HIV) infections.

Answer

Four distinct disease types are as follows:
1. HIV-associated gingivitis (HIV-G): A distinctive linear inflammation is seen around the gingival margin with possible punctate erythema extending throughout the width of the attached gingiva that may occur in the presence of excellent oral hygiene.
2. HIV-associated periodontitis (HIV-P): Characterized by rapid loss of attachment, connective tissue destruction and deep bone pain.
3. HIV-necrotizing gingivitis (HIV-NG).
4. Necrotizing stomatitis (NS): In this spontaneous sequestration of interdental bone along with extensive soft tissue necrosis occurs.

Since it was felt that the prefix 'HIV' was overdescriptive and caused potential, ethical and legal problems with confidentiality, the new classification has dropped the term HIV from individual disease titles:
 a. HIV-G has been changed to linear gingivitis.
 b. HIV-NG has been changed to necrotizing ulcerative gingivitis (NUG).
 c. HIV-P has been changed to necrotizing ulcerative periodontitis (NUP).
 d. Necrotizing stomatitis.

Q2. Enumerate the oral lesions associated with HIV infection.

Answer

Oral lesions associated with HIV infection		
Group I	*Group II*	*Group III*
Oral lesions strongly associated with HIV infection	Lesions less commonly associated with HIV infection	Lesions seen in HIV infection

1. Candidiasis
2. Hairy leukoplakia
3. Non-Hodgkin's lymphoma
4. Kaposi's sarcoma
5. Periodontal diseases
  • LGE: Linear gingival erythema
  • NUG: Necrotizing ulcerative gingivitis
  • NUP: Necrotizing ulcerative periodontitis
	1. Salivary gland diseases
	2. Melanotic hyperpigmentation
	3. Viral infection
	4. Bacterial infections
	5. Necrotizing stomatitis
		1. Recurrent aphthous stomatitis
		2. Osteomyelitis
		3. Sinusitis
		4. Fungal lesions other than candidiasis
		5. Cytomegalovirus infection
		6. Bacterial infections
		7. Exacerbation of apical periodontitis

CHAPTER 32

Diagnosis of Periodontal Diseases

Q1. What are the principles of diagnosis?

Answer

1. Sensitivity: Refers to the ability of a test or observation to detect the disease whenever it is present.
2. Specificity: Refers to the ability of a test or observation to clearly differentiate one disease from another.
3. Predictive value: Refers to the probability of the test results.

Q2. What are the stages of periodontal diagnosis?

Answer

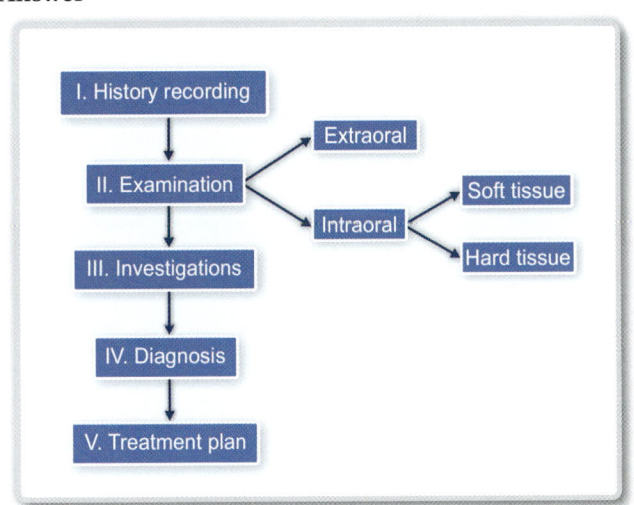

```
I. History recording
        ↓
II. Examination → Extraoral
                → Intraoral → Soft tissue
                            → Hard tissue
        ↓
III. Investigations
        ↓
IV. Diagnosis
        ↓
V. Treatment plan
```

Q3. Define the terms attrition, abrasion and erosion.

Answer

Attrition is the occlusal wear resulting from functional contacts with teeth and opposing teeth.

Abrasion refers to the loss of tooth substance induced by mechanical wear other than that of mastication.

Erosion is the wear to the non-occluding tooth surfaces, which is sharply defined wedge-shaped depression in the cervical area of the facial tooth surface.

Q4. What is fremitus test and mention its significance?

Answer

1. Class I: Mild vibrations detected and recorded as '+'.
2. Class II: Easily palpable vibrations, recorded as '++'.
3. Class III: Movements visible with naked eye and recorded as '+++'.

Significance: It is recorded to diagnose a case of trauma from occlusion by measuring the vibratory pattern of the teeth.

Q5. What are the causes of mobility?

Answer

Causes for mobility can be divided into local and systemic factors.

Local Factors

1. Bone loss and loss of tooth support:
   a. Bone destruction caused by extension of gingival inflammation, which can be either due to plaque products or pharmacologically active substances.
   b. Trauma from occlusion either in absence or associated with inflammation.
2. Hypofunction.
3. Periapical pathology.
4. After periodontal therapy.
5. Parafunctional habits like bruxism or clenching.
6. Pathology of jaws like tumor, cyst, etc.
7. Traumatic injury to dentoalveolar unit.
8. Tooth morphology.
9. Overjet and overbite.
10. Implant mobility.

Systemic Factors

1. Age.
2. Sex and race: Slightly higher incidence seen in females and Negros.

3. Menstrual cycle.
4. Oral contraceptives.
5. Pregnancy.
6. Systemic diseases such as Papillon-Lefevre syndrome, Down syndrome, neutropenia, Chediak-Higashi syndrome, etc.

CHAPTER 33

Prognosis

Q1. Define prognosis.
Answer

It is a prediction of the probable course, duration and outcome of a disease based on a general knowledge of the pathogenesis of the disease and the presence of risk factors for the disease.

Q2. Differentiate between prognosis and risk.
Answer

Differences between prognosis and risk	
Prognosis	*Risk*
It is the prediction of the duration, course and the termination of disease and its response to treatment	Deals with the likelihood that an individual will get a disease in a specified period
Prognostic factors are characteristics that predict the outcome of disease once the disease is present	Risk factors are those characteristics of an individual that put them at increased risk for getting a disease

Q3. Classify prognosis.
Answer

It is based on the factors to be considered, while determining the prognosis. The prognosis may be:
1. *Excellent prognosis:* No bone loss, excellent gingival condition, good patient cooperation, no systemic/environmental factors.
2. *Good prognosis:* One or more of the following: adequate remaining bone support, possibilities to control etiologic factors and establishes a maintainable dentition, adequate patient co-operation, no systemic/environmental factors or if present is well-controlled.
3. *Fair prognosis:* One or more of the following: less than adequate remaining bone support, some tooth mobility, grade I furcation involvement, adequate maintenance, acceptable patient cooperation, presence of limited systemic/environmental factors.
4. *Poor prognosis:* One or more of the following: moderate to advanced bone loss, tooth mobility, grade I and II furcation involvements, doubtful patient cooperation, difficult to maintain areas, presence of systemic/environmental factors.
5. *Questionable prognosis:* One or more of the following: advanced bone loss, grade II and III furcation involvements, tooth mobility, inaccessible areas, systemic/environmental factors.
6. *Hopeless prognosis:* One or more of the following: advanced bone loss, non-maintainable areas, extraction indicated, presence of uncontrolled systemic/environmental factors.

Q4. What are the factors determining prognosis?

Answer

```
                                Prognosis
        ┌───────────────┬──────────────┬──────────────┐
  Overall clinical  Systemic/        Local         Prosthetic/
     factors       Environmental    factors        Restorative
                      factors                        factors
   → Patient age   → Smoking      → Plaque/Calculus → Abutment selection
   → Disease       → Systemic     → Subgingival    → Caries
     severity       diseases        restorations
   → Plaque        → Genetic      → • Anatomic factors → Non-vital teeth
     control         factors         • Short, tapered roots
   → Patient       → Stress         • Enamel projections → Root resorption
     compliance                     • Enamel pearls
                                    • Bifurcation ridges
                                    • Root concavities
                                    • Developmental grooves
                                    • Root proximity
                                    • Furcation involvement
                                    • Tooth mobility
```

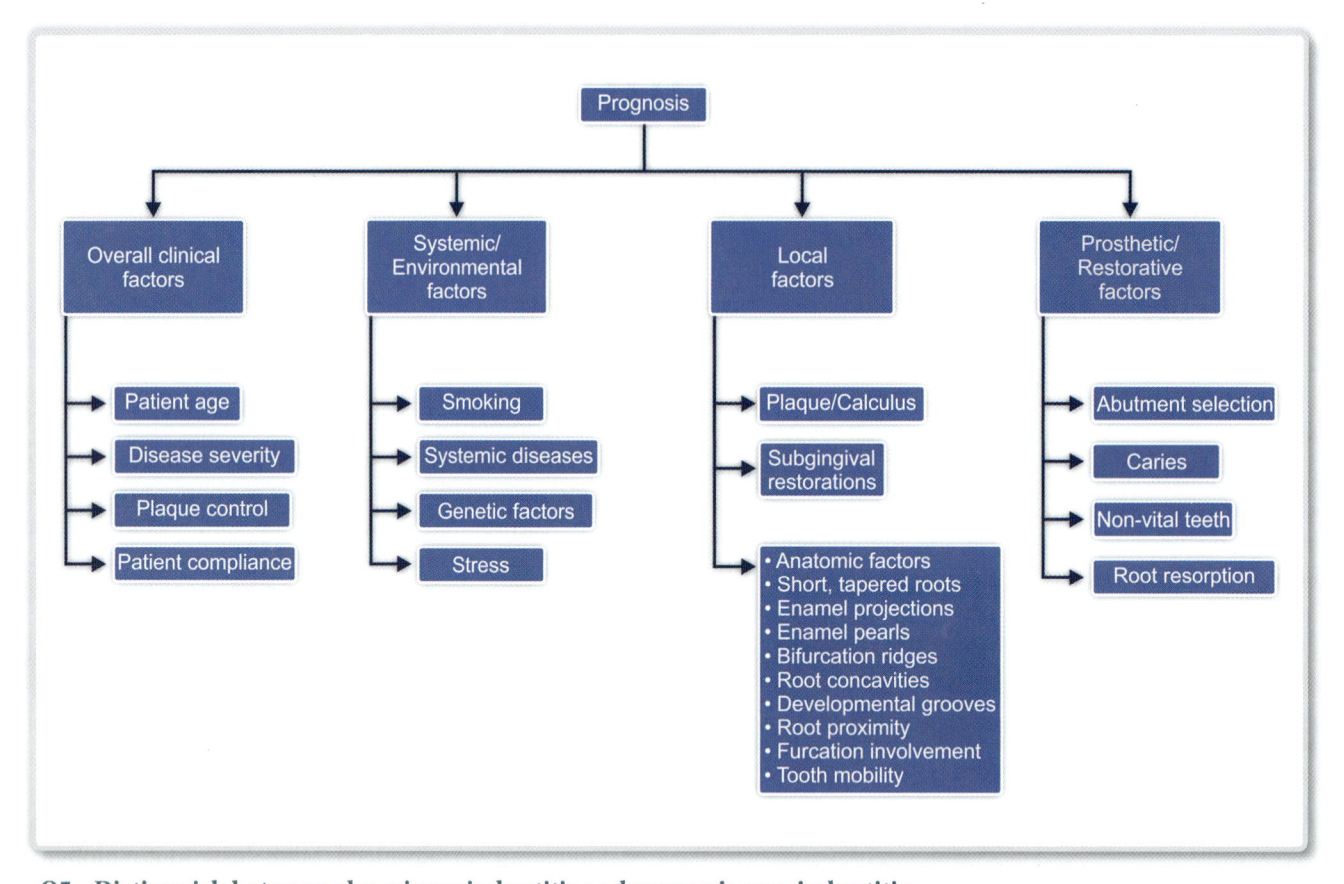

Q5. Distinguish between chronic periodontitis and aggressive periodontitis.

Answer

Distinction between chronic and aggressive periodontitis	
Chronic periodontitis	*Aggressive periodontitis*
Slowly progressive disease associated with local environmental factors.	Rapidly progressive disease with minimal/no local factors with increased level of *Aggregatibacter actinomycetemcomitans* and *Porphyromonas gingivalis*.
Can be localized or generalized.	Can be localized or generalized.
In case of not advanced attachment loss, prognosis is generally good. But inflammation has to be controlled through good oral hygiene and removal of local plaque-retentive factors.	Two common features are observed: a. Rapid attachment loss and bone destruction in an otherwise clinically healthy person. b. A familial aggregation.
In cases of severe disease with furcations involvement and increasing clinical mobility/who are non-compliant with oral hygiene, prognosis is downgraded from fair to poor.	Localized type, which occurs around the age of puberty and is localized to first molars and incisors, if diagnosed early can be treated conservatively with oral hygiene instructions and systemic antibiotic therapy. Resulting in excellent prognosis. In advanced cases, the prognosis is still good if the lesions are treated with debridement, local and systemic antibiotics and regenerative therapy.
	Generalized type, which is also seen in young patients with generalized interproximal attachment loss and poor antibody response. Secondarly aggravated by cigarette smoking does not respond well to conventional periodontal therapy, therefore prognosis is often fair, poor or questionable and the use of systemic antibiotics should be considered.

CHAPTER 34

Related Risk Factors Associated with Periodontal Diseases

Q1. Define risk.

Answer

Risk is the probability that an individual will develop a specific disease in a given period, which may vary from one individual to another. Risk assessment involves identifying elements that either may predispose a patient to developing periodontal disease or may influence progression of disease that already exists.

Q2. What are the risk factors of periodontal diseases?

Answer

1. *Tobacco smoking:* A direct relationship exists between smoking and prevalence of periodontal disease. Smoking has a negative impact on response to therapy.
2. *Diabetes:* It is a risk factor for periodontitis. Prevalence and severity is higher in diabetes than in those without diabetes.
3. Pathogenic bacteria and microbial tooth deposits:
   a. Quantity of plaque present on teeth is not of major importance. Composition or quality of the plaque biofilm is of importance.
   b. In terms of plaque, three specific bacteria have been identified as etiologic agents:
      - *Actinobacillus actinomycetemcomitans*
      - *Porphyromonas gingivalis*
      - *Bacteroides forsythus.*
4. *Anatomic factors:* Such as furcations, root concavities, developmental grooves, cervical enamel projections, enamel pearls and bifurcation ridges. All predispose to periodontitis, as they harbor bacterial plaque and present a challenge to clinician during instrumentation.

Q3. What are risk determinants or background characteristics?

Answer

It is defined as those risk factors that cannot be modified:

1. *Genetic factors:* It influences clinical measures of gingivitis probing pocket depth, attachment loss and interproximal bone height:
   a. A specific interleukin-1 (IL-1) genotype has been associated with severe chronic periodontitis.
   b. Immunologic alterations such as neutrophil abnormalities are under genetic control.
   c. Genetics plays a role in regulating the titer of protective IgG2 antibody response to *A. actinomycetemcomitans* in patients with aggressive periodontitis.
2. *Age:*
   a. Both the prevalence and severity of periodontal disease increases with age.
   b. Attachment loss and bone loss seen in elderly individuals is a result of prolonged exposure to other risk factors over a longer period of time.
   c. Changes related to old age such as intake of medications, decreased immune functions and altered nutritional status may increase susceptibility to periodontitis.
3. *Gender:* Males have more attachment loss than females and have a poorer oral hygiene; therefore more males are prone to periodontal diseases.
4. *Socioeconomic status:* Poor oral health is seen in lower socioeconomic status. This can be attributed to:
   a. Decreased dental awareness.
   b. Decreased dental visits.
5. *Stress:* Incidence of acute necrotizing ulcerative gingivitis (ANUG) increases during stressful situations:
   a. Emotional stress may interfere with normal immune.
   b. There is an apparent link between psychosocial factors and risk behavior such as smoking, poor oral hygiene and chronic periodontitis.
   c. Individuals with financial strain, distress, depression and inadequate coping mechanisms have more loss of attachment.

Q4. What are risk indicators of periodontal disease?

Answer

Risk indicators are probable or putative risk factors that have been identified in cross-sectional studies, but have not been confirmed through longitudinal studies.

Following are the risk indicators:
1. *HIV/acquired immunodeficiency syndrome:* It has been hypothesized that immune dysfunction associated with high HIV infection and AIDS increases the susceptibility to periodontal disease, though the evidence is not conclusive.
2. *Osteoporosis:* It does not initiate periodontitis by itself, there is reduced bone mass in osteoporosis and this may enhance the progression of periodontal disease.
3. *Infrequent dental visits:* Some studies have shown increased risk for severe periodontitis in patients who have not visited dentist for 3 or more years (although age factor also plays a role).

Q5. What are risk markers/predictors?

Answer

These are associated with increased risk for disease, but do not cause the disease. These factors also are identified in cross-sectional and longitudinal studies. A risk factor that can be used to predict the future course of disease is known as a risk marker:
1. Previous history of periodontal disease.
2. Bleeding on probing: Bleeding along with increased pocket depth may serve as an excellent predictor for future loss of attachment.

CHAPTER 35

Various Aids Including Advanced Diagnostic Aids

Q1. What are the aids used in clinical diagnosis in the field of periodontics?

Answer

1. Millimeter probe for gingival bleeding.
2. Measurement of gingival crevicular fluid flow with the help of a filter paper. Newer method is by use of a Periotron 6000.
3. Measurement of temperature by pressure-sensitive probes. Periotemp™ probe (Abiodent™).
4. Mouth odors—olfactometer.
5. Tooth mobility—mobilometer/periodontometer.
6. Periodontal screening and recording (PSR).

Q2. Enumerate various uses of probes.

Answer

1. To measure the pocket depth.
2. Quantification of bacterial plaque and gingival inflammation.
3. Determination of mucogingival relationship.
4. Measurement of gingival recession.
5. Location of calculus.
6. Identification of tooth irregularities.
7. Identification of tissue characteristics.
8. Determination of bleeding tendency.
9. Evaluation of bone support in the furcation areas of bifurcated and trifurcated teeth.

Q3. What are the various types of conventional periodontal probes?

Answer

1. Marquis color-coded probe: Calibrations are in 3 mm sections.
2. The University of North Carolina-15 probe (UNC-15): 15 mm long and markings are at 1 mm and color coding at the 5th, 10th and 15 mm.
3. The University of Michigan 'O' probe with Williams markings (at 1, 2, 3, 5, 7, 8, 9) 4 and 6 missing.
4. The Michigan 'O' probe with markings at 3, 6 and 8 mm.
5. The WHO probe, which has a 0.5 mm ball at the tip and millimeter markings at 3.5, 8.5 and 11.5 mm, and color coding from 3.5 to 5.5 mm.
6. Furcation areas can best be evaluated with the curved, blunt Nabers probe.

Q4. Classify periodontal probes.

Answer

First generation probes: Conventional, manual probes, e.g. conventional periodontal probes.

Second generation probes: The pressure-sensitive probes.

Third generation probes: Probes with controlled force application, automated measurements and computerized data capture.

Fourth generation: Records sequential probe positions along the gingival sulcus. They are still under research.

Fifth generation: Ultrasound probes, still under research.

Q5. Give examples of second generation probes.

Answer

Some of the examples of second generation probes are:
- Pressure probe (Vander Volden)
- Pressure sensitive probe (PSP)
- Borodontic probe
- Hunton probe (disposable probe)
- Yeaple probe (to assess dentinal hypersensitivity).

Q6. What are the limitations of conventional probes?

Answer

1. Probing depth obtained with periodontal probe does not coincide with the histological pocket depth, because the probe normally penetrates the coronal level of the junctional epithelium.
2. Reproducibility, which has been correlated with the variation in the probing force.

Q7. What are the limitations of all automated controlled force probes?

Answer

1. Reduced tactile sense of the operator.
2. Increased patient discomfort.
3. Presence or absence of inflammation often produced inaccurate measurement.

Q8. What are the features of probe used in periodontal screening and recording (PSR)?

Answer

It is designed for easier and faster screening and recording of the periodontal status of a patient or a group of population.

It uses a specially designed probe that has a 0.5 mm ball tip and is color-coded from 3.5 to 5.5 mm.

Q9. What are the instruments used to measure mobility?

Answer

Periodontometer and periotest.

Q10. What are the most commonly used radiographs in periodontal diagnosis?

Answer

The most commonly used radiographs in periodontal diagnosis are transmission radiographs. Transmission radiographs, including periapical and bitewing films are used to detect the amount of bone loss in any type of periodontitis. They should be used with less exposure to avoid any cervical burnout effect.

Q11. What are the disadvantages of conventional radiographs?

Answer

1. 30%–60% of the mineral content of the bone must be lost to visualize the change in the radiographic image, hence though very specific, lacks sensitivity.
2. Actual damage is more extensive than radiographs.
3. Radiographs are a two-dimensional representation of a three-dimensional anatomy.

Q12. How to minimize the radiographic distortion in dental office?

Answer

Techniques are available to minimize the radiographic distortion. First a long cone should be used (because parallel rays will minimize distortion).

Secondly, the use of parallel positioning devices helps to standardize the relationship between film, object and X-ray source, e.g. RINN XPR.

Disadvantage: Only a limited view of the osseous crest is available. Hence the use of extended cone projection instruments is recommended.

Q13. What are the advances in radiographic assessment?

Answer

Other Advanced Radiographic Aids

- Iodine-125 absorptiometry
- Photodensitometric analysis
- Digital radiography
- Substraction radiography
- Digital substraction radiography (DSR)
- Computer assisted densitometric image analysis (CADIA)
- Computerized tomography
- Nuclear medicine bone scan.

Q14. Enumerate the various microbiological aids used in periodontal diagnosis.

Answer

Because bacteria are the causative agents in periodontal diseases it makes sense to look for specific bacteria as indicators of disease activity.

Identification of Bacteria

1. Direct examination—microscopy:
   a. Light.
   b. Dark field.
2. Culture and sensitivity assay:
   a. Culture techniques:
      - Aerobic
      - Anaerobic.
   b. Speciation techniques:
      - Gas-liquid chromatography (GLC)
      - DNA homology.

Q15. What are the advantages and disadvantages of direct microscopy?

Answer

Advantages of direct microscopy: It is quick, easy and inexpensive means of screening a microbial sample for major morphotypes.

Disadvantages

- Inability to identify species
- Specimens have to be examined as soon as they are collected from the patients.

Q16. What are the different kinds of culture media?

Answer

Supportive media: Only allows growth of non-fastidious organisms.

CHAPTER 35 Various Aids Including Advanced Diagnostic Aids

Enriched media: Encourages the growth of organisms.

Non-selective media: Permits the growth of most oral microorganisms without specific inhibitory agents.

Selective media: Contains dyes, antibiotics that are inhibitory to all organisms except those being sought.

Q17. Enumerate different types of culture techniques.
Answer

1. Jar technique.
2. Pre-reduced anaerobic sterilized roll tubes (PRAS).
3. Anaerobic chamber techniques.
4. Enzyme reduction technique.

Q18. What is gas-liquid chromatography (GLC) and DNA probes?
Answer

1. *Gas-liquid chromatography:* In which various metabolic products of anaerobes are studied, which are unique enough to serve as markers for identification.
2. *DNA probes in the identification of periodontal pathogens:* It is based on the ability of DNA to hybridize or bind to the complementary strands of DNA having the exact base sequence.

Q19. Describe various immunological methods.
Answer

1. Immunofluorescence:
    - Direct immunofluorescence
    - Indirect immunofluorescence.
2. Enzyme-linked immunosorbent assay (ELISA).
3. Flow cytometry.
4. Latex agglutination.

Q20. What is biochemical diagnosis?
Answer

Byproducts of the cells (PMNLs), complement cleavage, e.g. C3, C4 in gingival crevicular fluid are studied.

Prostaglandins can differentiate between gingivitis and periodontitis, e.g. aggressive forms showed higher levels than chronic periodontitis. Active sites exhibited five-fold increase in PGE_2 levels than inactive sites. PGE_2 levels are studied by radioisotope assay (RIA).

Collagenase showed positive correlation with disease activity. It is studied by sodium dodecyl sulfate polyacrylamide gel electrophoresis (PAGE). In this they studied breakdown products resulting from incubation of collagen with gingival crevicular fluid.

Q21. What is PerioScan?
Answer

It is a diagnostic kit developed for identification of specific bacteria profile using an enzymatic reaction from plaque bacteria.

Q22. What is BANA test?
Answer

N-benzoyl-DL-arginine 2-naphthylamide (BANA) can identify:
- *Bacteroides forsythus*
- *Porphyromonas gingivalis* enzyme
- *Treponema denticola*
- *Capnocytophaga.*

These microorganisms have a common trypsin-like, which hydrolyzes the colorless substrate.

N-benzoyl-DL-arginine-2-naphthylamide—when hydrolysis takes place, it releases the chromophore beta-naphthylamide, which turns orange red when a drop of fast garnet is added to the solution.

Q23. What is filter separation enzyme immunoassay (FSEIA)?
Answer

It can identify *Aggregatibacter actinomycetemcomitans, Prevotella intermedia, P. gingivalis.* The clinician mixes the plaque sample taken with a paper point with this reagent to produce a colored reaction, which may be positive or negative. It requires 10–15 minutes of the office time.

CHAPTER 36

Treatment Plan

Q1. What is the importance of treatment plan?

Answer

The aim of the treatment plan is total treatment, i.e. coordination of all treatment procedures for the purpose of creating a well-functioning dentition in a healthy periodontal environment.

Q2. What are the four phases of treatment plan?

Answer

Preliminary phases or emergency phases are:
- Phase I therapy (etiotropic phase)
- Phase II therapy (surgical phase)
- Phase III therapy (restorative phase)
- Phase IV therapy (maintenance phase).

Q3. What all treatment procedures come under preliminary phase?

Answer

Treatment of emergencies:
- Dental or periapical abscess
- Periodontal abscess.
  Extraction of hopeless teeth and provisional replacement if needed.

Q4. What all procedures come under phase I therapy (etiotropic phase)?

Answer

- Plaque control
- Diet control
- Removal of calculus and root planing
- Correction of restorative and prosthetic irritational factors
- Excavation of caries and restorations (temporary or final)
- Antimicrobial therapy
- Occlusal therapy
- Minor orthodontic movement
- Provisional splinting.

Q5. What all procedures come under phase II therapy (surgical phase)?

Answer

- Periodontal surgery including placement of implants
- Root canal treatment.

Q6. What all procedures come under phase III therapy (restorative phase)?

Answer

- Final restorations
- Fixed and removable prosthesis
- Evaluation of response to restorative procedures
- Periodontal examination.

Q7. What all procedures come under phase IV therapy (maintenance phase)?

Answer

- Periodic recall visits
- Checking for plaque and calculus
- Gingival condition (pockets, inflammation)
- Occlusion, tooth mobility and other pathologic changes.

Q8. What is the preferred sequence of periodontal therapy?

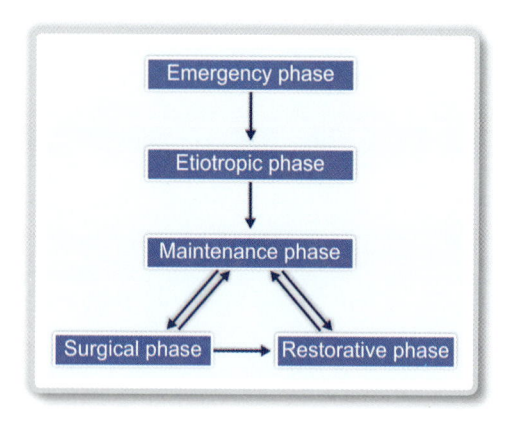

Answer

Emergency phase → Etiotropic phase → Maintenance phase ↔ Surgical phase → Restorative phase

CHAPTER 37

Rationale for Periodontal Treatment

Q1. Enumerate the factors affecting wound healing.

Answer

Local Factors

Healing is delayed due to contamination of microorganisms; irritation from plaque, food debris, necrotic tissue remnants and trauma from occlusion; excessive tissue manipulation during treatment and trauma to the tissues.

In addition, repetitive treatment procedures, which affect the orderly cellular activity in the healing process, topically applied cortisone and ionizing radiation can retard healing. Healing is improved by a local increase in temperature, debridement, immobilization of the healing area and pressure on the wound.

Systemic Factors

Healing is delayed in:
1. Older patients.
2. Generalized infections especially in patients with diabetes and other debilitating diseases.
3. By insufficient food intake, vitamin C deficiency, deficiency of proteins and other nutrients.
4. Increased levels of hormones such as cortisone.
5. Systemic stress, thyroidectomy, testosterone, adrenocorticotropic hormone and large doses of estrogen suppress the formation of granulation tissue and retard healing.

Q2. Define regeneration.

Answer

Regeneration is the biologic process by which the architecture and function of lost tissues are completely restored by formation of new periodontal ligament, alveolar bone and cementum.

Q3. Define repair.

Answer

Repair is the healing of tissues without completely restoring the lost tissues.

Q4. Define new attachment.

Answer

This is the reunion of connective tissue with a root surface that has been pathologically exposed.

Q5. Define reattachment.

Answer

This is the reunion of connective tissue and a root surface that have been separated by incision or injury.

Q6. What are four different sources of cells, which invade the surgical site during healing phase?

Answer

During healing, the area may be invaded by cells from four different sources:
1. Oral epithelium—results in long junctional epithelium.
2. Gingival connective tissue results in fibers parallel to root surface.
3. Bone cells—root resorption and ankylosis.
4. Only cells from periodontal ligament—results in new attachment.

CHAPTER 38

Periodontal Instrumentation

Q1. What are different parts of an instrument?
Answer

Periodontal instrument is composed of:
- Blade
- Shank
- Handle.

Q2. Classify periodontal instruments.
Answer

1. Diagnostic instruments: Probes and explorers.
2. Scaling, root planing and curettage instruments: These are classified as follows:
   a. For supragingival scaling:
      - Sickle scalers, cumine universal scaler, posterior Jacquette scaler, Morse scaler, surface scaler, cingulum scaler.
   b. For subgingival scaling:
      - Hoe scaler, chisel and file scalers are used to remove tenacious subgingival deposits
      - Curettes are used to plane the root surfaces by removing altered cementum and also for scraping the soft tissue wall of the pocket.
   c. Sonic and ultrasonic instruments.
3. Surgical instruments: Excisional and incisional instruments, surgical curettes and sickles, periosteal elevators, surgical chisels, hoes files, scissors and nippers.
4. Cleansing and polishing instruments:
   a. Rubber cups, brushes, dental tapes.
   b. Air-powder abrasive system.

Q3. What are different types of periodontal probes?
Answer

- Color-coded
- Non-color-coded.

Color-coded and Non-color-coded Probes

1. *The Marquis color-coded probe:* The calibrations are in 3 mm sections.
2. *The University of North Carolina-15 probe (UNC-15):* It is a 15 mm long probe with millimeter markings at each millimeter and color coding at the 5, 10 and 15 mm.
3. *Williams probe:* Has both color and non-color coding with markings at 1, 2, 3, 5, 7, 8, 9 and 10 mm.
4. *The Michigan 'O' probe with Williams marking:* At 1, 2, 3, 5, 7, 8, 9, 10 mm (4 and 6 are missing).
5. *The Michigan 'O' probe with markings:* At 3, 6, and 8 mm.
6. *The WHO probe:* It has a 0.5 mm ball at the tip and millimeter marking at 3.5, 8.5 and 11.5 mm and color coding from 3.5 to 5.5 mm.

Q4. What is the edge, shape and cross section of sickle scalers?
Answer

Sickle scalers have a flat surface and two cutting edges that converge in a sharply-pointed tip. The arch-shape of the instrument makes the tip so strong that it will not break off during use. They appear triangular in cross section. The sickle scaler is inserted under ledges of calculus no more than 1 mm below the gingival sulcus. It is used with a pull stroke.

Q5. What are the uses of curettes?
Answer

The curette is the instrument of choice for removing deep subgingival calculus, altered cementum, for root planing and for removing the soft tissue lining the periodontal pocket.

Curette can be adapted to provide good access to deep pockets, with minimal soft tissue trauma. There are cutting edges on both sides of the blade.

Q6. How are curettes classified?

Answer

There are two basic types of curettes:
1. Universal.
2. Area-specific.

Q7. Difference between universal and area specific curettes.

Answer

Distinction between Gracey and universal curettes		
Features	Gracey curette	Universal curette
Area of use	Set of many curettes designed for specific areas and surfaces	One curette designed for all areas and surfaces
Cutting edge	One cutting edge used, work is done with the outer edge only	Both cutting edges used, work is done with outer or inner edge
Curvature	Curved in two planes, blade curves up and to the side	Curved in one plane, blades curves up and not to the side
Blade angle	Offset blade, face of blade beveled at 60 degrees to the shank	Not offset, face of blade beveled at 90 degrees to the shank

Q8. Name some universal curettes.

Answer

Barnhart curettes No. 1-2 and 5-6 and Columbia curettes No. 13-14, 2R-2L and 4R-4L. Other universal curettes include Younger-Good No. 7-8, the McCalls No. 17-18 and Indiana University No. 17-18.

Q9. Name some area specific curettes.

Answer

1. Double-ended Gracey curettes.
2. Extended shank curettes or After Five curettes.
3. Langer and Mini Langer curettes.

Q10. What are the standard Gracey instrument series? Where it is used?

Answer

- Gracey No. 1-2 and 3-4: For anterior teeth
- Gracey No. 5-6: For anterior teeth and premolars
- Gracey No. 7-8 and 9-10: Posterior teeth; facial and lingual
- Gracey No. 11-12: Posterior teeth; mesial
- Gracey No. 13-14: Posterior teeth; distal.
  Recent additions to Gracey set are:
- Gracey No. 15-16 and No. 17-18: No. 15-16 is a modification of No. 11-12; No. 17-18 is a modification of No. 13-14. It has a shank elongated by 3 mm.

Q11. What are extended shank curettes or After Five curettes?

Answer

Hu-Friedy After Five curettes are modifications of the standard Gracey curette design. The shank is 3 mm longer, allowing extension into deeper periodontal pockets of 5 mm or more, other features include a thinned blade for smoother subgingival insertion or reduced tissue distention with a large diameter, tapered shank.

All the standard Gracey numbers except No. 9-10 are available in the After Five series.

Q12. What are mini-bladed curettes?

Answer

They are modifications of After Five curettes. The shorter blade allows easier insertion and adaptation in deep, narrow pockets, furcations, developmental grooves, line angles and deep, tight, facial, lingual or palatal pockets.

As with the After Fives, the Mini Fives are available in all standard Gracey number except for the No. 9-10.

Q13. What are Langer and Mini Langer curettes?

Answer

This set of 3 curettes combines the shank design of the standard Gracey No. 5-6, 11-12 and 13-14 curettes with a universal blade honed at 90 degrees rather than the offset blade of the Gracey curette. Hence, these curettes offer a blend of both Gracey and universal curette and can be adapted both on the mesial and distal surfaces without changing instruments.

Q14. What are the instruments designed for the retrieval of broken instrument tips from the periodontal pocket?

Answer

Schwartz periotrievers: They are a set of two double-ended, highly magnetized instruments.

Q15. What are hoe scalers?

Answer

They are used for scaling ledges or rings of calculus. The blade is bent at a 99 degree angle; the cutting edge is beveled at 45 degrees. The hoe scalers are used in the following manner:

1. The blade is inserted to the base of the periodontal pocket, so that it makes a two point contact with the tooth. This stabilizes the instrument and prevents nicking of the tooth.

2. The instrument is activated with a firm pull stroke toward the crown, with every effort being made to preserve the two point contact with the tooth.

Q16. Name some hoe scalers.
Answer

McCalls hoe scalers No. 3, 4, 5, 6, 7 and 8 are a set of six hoe scalers designed to provide access to all the tooth surfaces.

Q17. What are periodontal files and its function?
Answer

They have a series of blades on a base. Their primary function is to fracture or crush tenacious calculus. Files can easily gouge and roughen root surfaces when used improperly. Therefore they are not suitable for fine scaling and root planing. They are sometimes used for removing overhanging margins of dental restorations.

Q18. What are the chisel scalers?
Answer

Usually used in the proximal surfaces of anterior teeth (too closely spaced). It is a double-ended instrument with a curved shank at one end and a straight shank at the other. The instrument is activated with a push motion.

Q19. What are Quéntin furcation curettes?
Answer

These are the curettes specifically designed to fit into the roof or floor of the furcation. These curettes are nothing, but hoe scalers with a shallow, half moon radius and the tip is curved in such a way that it also fits into the developmental depressions.

Q20. Name the types of ultrasonic and sonic instruments.
Answer

Two types of ultrasonic units are:
1. *Magnetostrictive:* Vibration of the tip is elliptical; hence all the sides can be used.
2. *Piezoelectric:* Pattern of vibration of the tip is linear; only two sides of the tip are active.

Q21. What is the range of frequency of ultrasonic vibrations?
Answer

Ultrasonic vibrations range from 20,000 to 45,000 cycles/second. They operate in a wet field and have attached water outlets.

Q22. What is dental endoscope?
Answer

It is introduced for use subgingivally, in the diagnosis, treatment of periodontal diseases. Produced by Dentalview Inc and called the perioscopy system.

It consists of reusable fiberoptic endoscope over which there is a sterile sheath. The fiberoptic endoscope fits onto the periodontal probes and ultrasonic instruments that have been designed to accept it.

Q23. What is the ethylene vinyl acetate (EVA) system?
Answer

They are most efficient and least traumatic instruments, for correcting overhanging or overcontoured proximal alloy and resin restorations.

Q24. What are different cleansing and polishing instruments?
Answer

- Rubber cups
- Bristle brushes
- Dental tape
- Air-powder polishing.

Q25. What is Prophy-Jet?
Answer

A specially designed hand piece that delivers air powdered slurry of warm water and sodium bicarbonate, this instrument is called Prophy-Jet. It is effective for the removal of extrinsic stains and soft deposits.

Q26. What are the types of sharpening stones?
Answer

Ceramics, Arkansas, India stone, Nievart whitten (steel).

Q27. Name some automatic sharpening instruments.
Answer

- PerioStar 2000
- PerioStar 3000.

Q28. Enumerate excisional and incisional instruments.
Answer

1. Periodontal knives (gingivectomy knives): For example, Kirkland knife.
2. Interdental knives: For example, Orban knife No. 1-2, Merrifield knife No. 1, 2, 3 and 4.
3. Surgical blades: For example, No. 12D, 15 and 15C.

4. Electrosurgery (radiosurgery) techniques and instrumentation:
   a. Electrosection used for incisions, excisions and tissue planing.
   b. Electrocoagulation, coagulation or hemorrhage control.
   c. Electrofulguration not in general use in dentistry.
   d. Electrodesiccation not in general use in dentistry.

Q29. What is the use of surgical curettes and sickles?

Answer

Surgical curettes and sickles: Required for the removal of granulation tissue, fibrous interdental tissue and tenacious subgingival deposits. For example:
- Kramer curettes No. 1, 2, 3 and Langer curettes
- Kirkland surgical instruments
- Ball scaler No. B2-B3.

Q30. What is the use of surgical chisels and hoes?

Answer

They are used during periodontal surgery for removing and reshaping bone.

Chisels are used with a push stroke whereas surgical hoes are used with a pull stroke. For example:
- Ochsenbein No. 1-2, chisel
- Rhodes chisel.

Q31. What is the use of surgical files in periodontal surgery?

Answer

They are used primarily to smoothen rough, bony, ledges and to remove all areas of necrotic bone. For example, Schluger and Sugarman files.

Q32. What is the use of scissors and nippers?

Answer

Scissors and nippers used for removing tabs of tissue during gingivectomy, trimming the margins of flaps, enlarging incisions in periodontal abscesses and removing muscle attachments in mucogingival surgery. For example, Goldman-Fox No. 16 scissors.

CHAPTER 39

Principles of Periodontal Instrumentation Including Scaling and Root Planing

Q1. What are the general principles of instrumentation?

Answer

1. Accessibility (positioning of patient and operator).
2. Visibility, illumination and retraction.
3. Condition of instruments (sharpness).
4. Maintaining a clean field.
5. Instrument stabilization.

Q2. What should be the ideal clinician position?

Answer

Neutral Seated Position for the Clinician

1. Forearm parallel to the floor.
2. Weight evenly balanced.
3. Thighs parallel to the floor.
4. Hip angle of 90 degrees.
5. Seat height positioned low enough so that the heels of your feet touch the floor.
6. When working from clock positions 9:00–12:00, spread feet apart so that your legs and the chair base form a tripod, which creates a stable position.
7. Avoid positioning your legs under the back of the patient's chair.
8. Back straight and the head erect.

Q3. What is ideal patient position?

Answer

The patient should be in a supine position and placed in such a way that the mouth is close to the resting elbow of the clinician.

Body: The patient's heels should be slightly higher than the tip of his or her nose. The back of the chair should be nearly parallel to the floor for maxillary treatment areas. The chair back may be raised slightly for mandibular treatment areas.

Head: The foremost of the patient's head should be even with the upper edge of the headrest:
- For mandibular areas—chin down position
- For maxillary areas—chin up position.

Headrest: If the headrest is adjustable, it should be raised or lowered, so that the patient's neck and head are aligned with the torso.

Q4. Describe the ideal clinical positions for right- and left-handed clinicians.

Answer

Clinical positions for right- and left-handed clinicians	
Right-handed clinician	Left-handed clinician
7 O'clock position, to the front of the patient's head	5 O'clock position, to the front of the patient's head
9 O'clock position, to the side of the patient's head	3 O'clock position, to the side of the patient's head
10–11 O'clock, to the back of the patient's head	2–10 O'clock position, to the back of the patient's head
12 O'clock position, directly behind the patient's head	12 O'clock position, directly behind the patient's head

Q5. What are the types of mouth mirror surfaces?

Answer

Various Types of Mirror Surfaces

- Front surface:
  - Produces clean clear image with no distortion
  - Good image quality
  - Easily scratchable.
- Concave surface:
  - Image is magnified
  - Distortion of the image.
- Plane (flat surface):
  - Produces double image
  - Double image is distracting.

Q6. What are the various uses of a dental mirror?

Answer

1. Indirect vision.
2. Retraction.
3. Indirect illumination.
4. Transillumination.

Q7. What is transillumination?

Answer

When transilluminating a tooth, the mirror is used to reflect light through the tooth surface. The transilluminated-tooth almost will appear to glow. It is effective only with anterior teeth because they are thin enough to allow the light to pass through them.

Q8. How retraction is achieved?

Answer

Retraction provides visibility, accessibility and illumination. The following methods are effective for retraction:

1. Use of the mirror to deflect the cheek while the fingers of the non-operating hand retract the lips and protect the angle of the mouth from irritation by the mirror handle.
2. Use of the mirror alone to retract the lips and cheek.
3. Use of fingers of the non-operating hand to retract the lips.
4. Use of the mirror to retract the tongue.
5. Combination of the preceding methods.

While retracting, care should be taken to avoid irritation to the angles of the mouth.

Q9. Why sharpening of an instrument is required?

Answer

The working ends of pointed or bladed instruments must be sharp to be effective.

Advantages of Sharpness

1. Easier calculus removal.
2. Improved stroke control.
3. Reduced number of strokes.
4. Increased patient comfort.
5. Reduced clinician fatigue.

Ideally, it is best to sharpen your instruments after autoclaving and then reautoclave them prior to patient treatment. Dull instruments may lead to incomplete calculus removal and unnecessary trauma because of excess force applied.

Q10. What is the importance of a clean operative field? How we can achieve it?

Answer

Instrumentation can be hampered if the operative field is obscured by saliva, blood and debris. Adequate suction is essential and can be achieved with a saliva ejector or an aspirator:

1. Blood and debris can be removed from the operative field with suction and by wiping or blotting with gauze squares.
2. The operative field should also be flushed occasionally with water.
3. Compressed air and gauze square can be used to facilitate visual inspection of tooth surfaces just below the gingival margin during instrumentation.
4. Retractable tissue can also be deflected away from the tooth by gently packing the edge of gauze square into the pocket with the back of a curette.

Q11. Why instrument stabilization is essential?

Answer

Stability of the instrument and the hand is the primary requisite for controlled-instrumentation. Stability and control is essential for effective instrumentation and to avoid injury to the patient or clinician.

Q12. What are the two factors that guide the stability of an instrument?

Answer

The two factors that provide stability are instrument grasp and finger rest.

Q13. What are different types of grasps?

Answer

Pen grasp: The typical way of holding pen or pencil.

Modified pen grasp: The most effective and stable grasp for all periodontal instruments. This grasp allows precise control of the working end, permits a wide range of movements and facilitates good tactile conduction.

Palm and thumb grasp: It is useful for stabilizing instruments during sharpening and for manipulating air and water syringes.

Q14. What is correct finger placement for stabilizing the instrument?

Answer

Digit	Recommended position and function
Thumb and index	The finger pads rest opposite to each other at or near the junction of the handle and the shank. They do not overlap and a tiny space exists between them. The instrument is held in a relaxed manner. The index finger and thumb curve outward from the handle in a C-shape. The main function of these digits is to hold the instrument.
Middle	One side of the finger pad rests lightly on the instrument shank. The other side of the finger pad rests against the ring finger. It helps to guide the working end and also feel the vibration.

Contd...

Contd...

Digit	Recommended position and function
Ring	Fingertip balances firmly on the tooth to support the weight of the hand and instrument. The finger is held straight and upright to act as a strong support beam for the hand.
Little	It should be held in a relaxed manner with no function.

Q15. What is the significance of good finger rest? Which finger is preferred?

Answer

The finger rest serves to stabilize the hand and the instrument by providing a firm fulcrum, as movements are made to activate the instrument. A good finger rest prevents injury and laceration of the gingival and surrounding tissues.

The ring finger is preferred by most clinicians for the finger rest. Maximal control is achieved when the middle finger is kept between the instrument shank and the fourth finger. This built-up fulcrum is an integral part of the wrist-forearm action that activates the powerful working stroke for calculus removal.

Q16. How finger rests are classified?

Answer

Finger rests may be generally classified as intraoral finger rests or extraoral fulcrums.

Q17. What are the advantages of standard intraoral finger rests?

Answer

The finger rests on a stable tooth surface immediately adjacent to the working area.

Advantages

1. Provides the most stable, secured support for the hand.
2. Provides leverage and power for instrumentation.
3. Provides excellent tactile transfer to the fingers.
4. Permits precise stroke control.
5. Allows forceful stroke pressure with the least amount of stress to the hand and fingers.
6. Decreases the likelihood of injury to the patient.

Q18. What are the disadvantages of standard intraoral finger rests?

Answer

1. May not be practical for use in edentulous areas.
2. May be difficult to obtain parallelism of the lower shank to the tooth surface for accessing deep pockets.

Q19. Name advanced intraoral finger rests.

Answer

1. Modified intraoral fulcrum.
2. Piggy-backed fulcrum.
3. Cross-arch fulcrum.
4. Opposite arch fulcrum.
5. Finger-on-finger fulcrum.

Q20. What is modified intraoral fulcrum?

Answer

It is achieved by combining an altered modified pen grasp with a standard intraoral fulcrum. It is useful while instrumenting the maxillary teeth. It alters the point of contact between the middle and ring fingers in the grasp.

Advantages: As follows:

1. Provides good stable support for the clinician's hand.
2. Provides leverage, strength and good stroke control.
3. Provides good tactile sensitivity to clinician's finger.
4. Improves access to deep pockets on maxillary teeth and facilitates parallelism of lower shank to proximal root surfaces.

Disadvantage: Requires more muscle control.

Q21. What is piggy-backed fulcrum?

Answer

The middle finger rests on top of the ring finger.

Advantages: As follows:

1. Improved access to mandibular posterior aspects away from the clinician.
2. Enhances the whole hand working together as a unit.

Disadvantage: In patients with limited opening it cannot be used.

Q22. What is cross-arch fulcrum?

Answer

It is accomplished by resting the ring finger on a tooth on the opposite side of the arch from the teeth being instrumented.

Advantage: Allows improved access to the lingual aspect of mandibular posterior teeth.

Disadvantage: Decreases tactile sensitivity and makes strokes difficult.

Q23. What is opposite arch fulcrum?

Answer

It is accomplished by resting the ring finger on the opposite arch.

Advantage: Facilitates access to deep pockets.

Disadvantages: As follows:
1. Decreases tactile information.
2. Uncomfortable for patients with temporomandibular joint (TMJ) problems.

Q24. What is finger-on-finger fulcrum?

Answer

It is accomplished by resting the ring finger on the index finger.

Advantages: As follows:
1. Provides stable rest to fulcrum finger.
2. Improves access to deep pockets.

Disadvantage: Non-dominant hand cannot be used for retraction or to hold the mirror.

Q25. What is basic extraoral fulcrum?

Answer

They are essential for effective instrumentation of some aspects of maxillary posterior teeth:
1. *Knuckle-rest technique or palm up technique:* The clinician rests the knuckle against the patients chin or cheek.
2. *Chin-cup technique or palm down technique:* The clinician cups the patients chin with the palm of the hand.

Advantage: Facilitates instrumentation of the proximal root surfaces of maxillary molars.

Disadvantages: As follows:
1. Least effective of all fulcrum techniques.
2. Stroke control is more difficult and decreases tactile information.

Q26. Define instrument adaptation.

Answer

Adaptation refers to the manner in which the working end of a periodontal instrument is placed against the surface of a tooth. The object of adaptation is to make the working end of the instrument conform to the contour of the tooth surface.

Q27. What is meant by angulation?

Answer

It refers to the angle between the face of a bladed instrument and the tooth surface.

Q28. What should be the face to tooth surface angulation for insertion beneath the gingival margin?

Answer

Between 0 and 40 degrees.

Q29. What is the ideal tooth-blade angulation for calculus removal?

Answer

For calculus removal, angulation should be between 45 and 90 degrees. The exact blade angulation depends on the amount and nature of calculus, the procedure being performed and condition of tissue during scaling or root planing, with angulation of less than 45 degrees, the cutting edge will slide over the calculus smoothening or burnishing it.

Q30. What is the ideal tooth-blade angulation for gingival curettage?

Answer

When gingival curettage is indicated, angulation greater than 90 degrees is deliberately established.

Q31. What is meant by lateral pressure?

Answer

It refers to the pressure created when force is applied against the surface of a tooth with the cutting edge of a bladed instrument. Exact amount of pressure depends upon the procedure performed. It may be firm, moderate or light when insufficient lateral pressure is applied rough ledges or lumps may be shaved to thin, smooth sheets of burnished calculus.

Q32. Why repeated application of excessively heavy strokes should be avoided?

Answer

Repeated application of excessively heavy strokes will nick or gouge the root surface. The careful application of varied and controlled amounts of lateral pressure during instrumentation is an integral part of effective scaling and root planing techniques.

Q33. What are the different types of strokes?

Answer

There are four types of strokes:
1. Placement stroke.
2. Exploratory stroke or assessment stroke.
3. Scaling stroke.
4. Root planing stroke.

Q34. What is placement stroke?

Answer

The placement stroke is used to position the working end of an instrument apical to a calculus deposit or at the base of a sulcus or pocket.

Q35. What are the characteristics of different types of strokes?
Answer

	Assessment stroke	Calculus removal/Scaling stroke	Root planing stroke
Purpose	Assess tooth—anatomy, level of attachment Detect calculus and other plaque retentive factors	Remove calculus deposits	Remove residual calculus, bacterial plaque and byproducts
Used with	Probes/explorers, curettes	Sickle scalers, curettes, files	Curettes
Insertion	0–40 degrees	0–40 degrees	0–40 degrees
Working angulation	50–70 degrees	70–80 degrees	60–70 degrees
Lateral pressure	Contacts tooth surface, but no pressure applied	Moderate to firm scraping	Light to moderate
Character	Fluid stroke of moderate length	Powerful strokes short in length	Lighter strokes of moderate length
Direction	Vertical, oblique, horizontal	Vertical, oblique, horizontal	Vertical, oblique, horizontal
Number	Many, covering entire root surface	Limited, to area where needed	Many, covering entire root surface

Q36. What are the different types of stroke directions?
Answer

Instrument strokes are initiated using a pull stroke in a coronal direction away from the junctional epithelium.

Pull strokes may be made in vertical, oblique or horizontal directions.

Vertical strokes: Facial, lingual, proximal surfaces of anterior teeth, mesial and distal surfaces of posterior teeth.

Oblique strokes: Facial and lingual surfaces of anterior and posterior teeth.

Horizontal strokes or circumferential strokes: Line angles of posterior teeth, furcation areas.

Q37. Define scaling.
Answer

This is the process by which plaque and calculus are removed from both supragingival and subgingival tooth surfaces.

Q38. Define root planing.
Answer

This is the process by which residual embedded calculus and portions of cementum are removed from the roots to produce a smooth, hard, clean surface.

Q39. What is the prime objective of scaling and root planing?
Answer

The prime objective of scaling and root planing is to restore gingival health by completely removing the tooth surface elements that provoke gingival inflammation.

Q40. What are the two basic types of curettes?
Answer
- Universal
- Gracey.

Q41. What is the principle of working of universal curettes?
Answer

Universal Curettes

The working ends of the universal curettes are designed in pairs so that all surfaces of the teeth can be treated with one-double ended instrument or a matched pairs of single-ended instruments. In any given quadrant, one end of universal curette will adapt to the mesial surface and the other end to the distal surface. The end that adapts to the mesial surface of the facial aspects also adapts to the distal surface on the lingual aspect and vice versa.

Q42. What is the principle of working of Gracey curettes?
Answer

Gracey Curettes

1. Determine the cutting edge by visually inspecting the blade and confirmed by lightly adapting the chosen cutting edge to the tooth with the lower shank parallel to the surface of the tooth.
2. Make sure the lower shank is parallel to the surface to be instrumented.
3. When using intraoral finger rests, keep the fourth and middle fingers together in a built-up fulcrum for maximum control and wrist-arm action.
4. Use extraoral fulcrum or mandibular finger rests for optimal angulation when working on the maxillary posterior teeth.
5. Concentrate on using the cutting edge (lower) for calculus removal.
6. Allow the wrist and forearm to carry the burden of the stroke, rather than flexing the fingers.
7. Roll the handle slightly between the thumb and fingers to keep the blade adapted as the working end is advanced around line angles and into concavities.

8. Module lateral pressure from firm to moderate to light depending on the nature of calculus.

Q43. What is the working principle of ultrasonic scalers?

Answer

Ultrasonic devices work by converting electrical current to mechanical energy in the form of high frequency vibration of instrument tip.

Q44. What is the range of frequency at which sonic and ultrasonic scalers work?

Answer

They operate at frequencies 18,000–50,000 cycles/second whereas sonic scalers need 2,000–6,500 cycles/second.

Q45. What are the two types of ultrasonic scalers?

Answer

Two types of ultrasonic units are magnetostrictive and piezoelectric units.

Q46. What are the benefits of water lavage obtained during ultrasonic scaling?

Answer

The water lavage has three benefits on the treatment site:
1. *Flushing action:* Flushes calculus, blood, bacteria, plaque from treatment site.
2. *Cavitation:* As the water exits from instrument tip, it forms a spray of tiny bubbles that collapses and releases shock waves in a process known as cavitation. It causes lysis of bacterial cell wall.
3. *Acoustic streaming:* The continuous stream of water produces tremendous pressure within the confined space of periodontal pocket. This effect is called acoustic streaming. Bacteria, gram-negative rods are sensitive to acoustic streaming.

Q47. What are the uses of ultrasonic and sonic instrumentation?

Answer

Treating Periodontal Disease
1. Debridement of calculus, plaque.
2. Removing overhanging restorations.
3. Improved access to furcation.
4. Increased patient comfort.
5. Reduced amount of time, a benefit for both patient and dentist.

Q48. What are dental aerosols?

Answer

Dental procedures produce airborne particles called aerosols, into surrounding environment. These aerosols contain microorganisms, blood, saliva and oral debris.

Microorganisms can survive up to 24 hours. Hence, patient should rinse with antimicrobial solution prior to treatment. Laminar airflow system, which filters the organisms in air, is recommended.

Q49. What are the contraindications of ultrasonic instruments?

Answer

Contraindications

Use of ultrasonic instruments is contraindicated in patients with:
1. Cardiac pacemaker.
2. Communicable disease.
3. Respiratory disease or difficulty in breathing.
4. With compromised gag reflex or difficulty in swallowing.
5. With porcelain crown, titanium dental implants, composite resin-restoration, demineralized enamel surface or dentinal hypersensitivity.
6. In children: Vibrations may damage growing tissue. Newly-erupted and primary teeth have large pulp chamber that are more susceptible to heat generated by instruments.

CHAPTER 40

Plaque Control

Q1. What is the definition of plaque control?

Answer

It is the removal of microbial plaque and the prevention of its accumulation on the teeth and adjacent gingival surfaces.

Q2. What are the goals of plaque control measures?

Answer

1. Plaque control retards the formation of calculus.
2. Removal of plaque leads to resolution of gingival inflammation.
3. Good plaque control facilitates return to and preservation of oral health.

Q3. What are the basic approaches for plaque control?

Answer

There are two basic approaches for plaque control:
1. Mechanical:
    a. Individual.
    b. Professional—for subgingival plaque control, e.g. scaling and root planing.
2. Chemical:
    a. Individual.
    b. Professional.

Q4. What are the various cleaning aids used by an individual for mechanical plaque control?

Answer

Individual mechanical plaque control is achieved by:
1. Toothbrush: Manual or powered.
2. Interdental aids:
    a. Dental floss:
        i. Unwaxed.
        ii. Waxed.
    b. Triangular toothpicks:
        i. Handheld.
        ii. Proxa-pic.
    c. Brushes: Proxabrush, bottlebrushes.
    d. Yarns, gauze strips, pipe cleaners.
3. Others:
    a. Rubber tip stimulator.
    b. Water irrigators.

Q5. What are the ADA specifications of a toothbrush?

Answer

ADA specifications of a toothbrush: The head of the brush should be:
1. 1–1¼ inches long.
2. 2–4 rows of bristles.
3. 5/16 to 3/8 inches wide.
4. 5–12 tufts per row.
5. 80–86 bristles per tuft.

Q6. Describe the design of a toothbrush.

Answer

A toothbrush consists of handle, shank and head. It has bristles, which when bunched together are called tufts. The extreme end of the head is toe and that close to the handle is the heel.
1. Size: Large, medium and small.
2. Lateral profile: Flat, convex, concave and scalloped.

Q7. Why nylon bristles are preferred over natural (hog) bristles?

Answer

Two types of bristles are available, nylon (synthetic) and natural (hog). Nylon bristles are preferred. Natural bristles are more susceptible to breakage and fraying, contamination with bacteria is high.

Q8. What are the factors responsible for hardness of a bristles?

Answer

Hardness: Depends on material, diameter and length:
1. Nylon bristles are more flexible.
2. Soft: 0.007–0.009 inches (No. 7, 8, 9).
3. Medium: 0.010–0.012 inches (No. 10, 11, 12).
4. Hard: 0.013–0.014 inches (No. 13, 14).
5. Extra hard: 0.015 inches (No. 15).

If the bristles are soft, they should be set close. If they are hard they should be more widely spaced.

Q9. What is the recommended frequency of brushing?

Answer

1. Frequency of brushing: Every 12 hours.
2. Frequency of change of brush: Every 3 months.

Q10. What should be the time duration for brushing?

Answer

Length of brushing time: Initially 10–20 minutes is required until the patient becomes more precise. Later 3–5 minutes may suffice.

Q11. Enumerate various brushing techniques.

Answer

According to brushing motions used in brushing techniques:
1. Horizontal:
   a. Reciprocating (scrub).
2. Vibratory:
   a. Bass method.
   b. Stillman's method.
   c. Charter's method.
3. Vertical sweeping:
   a. Rolling stroke.
   b. Modified bass.
   c. Modified stillman's.
   d. Leonard.
   e. Smith-Bell (physiological technique).
4. Rotary (Fones) technique.

Q12. What is the other name of Bass method?

Answer: It is also called intrasulcular method.

Q13. What are the advantages of Bass method?

Answer

1. Short 'back and forth' motion is easy to master.
2. Cleaning action is concentrated on the cervical and interproximal portions of the teeth, where most of the dental plaque detrimental to the gingiva is located.

Q14. What is the modification in modified Bass method?

Answer

The first part of the modified Bass method is identical to the Bass method. The modification consists of sweeping the bristles downwards over the tooth surface occlusally after completing the vibratory motion in the gingival sulci.

Q15. Describe Stillman's method of toothbrushing.

Answer

Stillman's Method

With Stillman's technique, the bristle ends are placed at a 45° angle, with the bristles placed partly on the gingiva and partly on the cervical portion of the teeth.

Once the bristles are in place, pressure is applied to blanch the gingiva and a gentle, but firm vibratory rotary motion is applied to the brush with the bristles remaining in the same position.

Advantage

It removes soft deposits from cervical areas.

Q16. What is the modified Stillman's technique?

Answer

1. The soft or medium, multitufted brush should be placed with the bristle ends resting partly on the cervical portion of the teeth and partly on the adjacent gingiva, pointing in an apical position, directed at an oblique angle to the long axis of the teeth.
2. Pressure is applied laterally against the gingival margin to produce a perceptible blanching.
3. The brush is activated with 20 short 'back and forth' strokes and is simultaneously moved in a coronal direction along the attached gingiva, the gingival margin and tooth surface. This process is repeated on all the teeth.

To reach lingual surfaces of the maxillary and mandibular incisors, the handle of the brush is held in a vertical position, engaging heel of the brush. With this technique the sides rather than the ends of the bristles are used, penetration of the bristles into gingival sulci is avoided.

Q17. What is the advantage of modified Stillman's technique?

Answer

Advantages

The modified Stillman method may be recommended for cleaning areas with progressing gingival recession and root exposure to prevent abrasive tissue destruction.

Q18. Describe Charter's method.

Answer

The Charter's method is as given below:
1. A soft or medium, multitufted brush is placed on the tooth with bristles pointing toward the crown at a 45° angle to long axis of the teeth.
2. The sides of bristles are flexed against the gingiva and the 'back and forth' vibratory motion is used to massage the gingiva.

Q19. What are the advantages of Charter's method?

Answer

This method is effective particularly in cases with receded interdental papillae, it is suitable for gentle plaque removal and gingival massage, when using soft brush and this technique can be recommended for temporary cleaning in areas of healing wounds after periodontal surgery.

Q20. What is roll technique/Fones method?

Answer

Technique: The bristles are first directed apically and then swept in an occlusal direction with a rolling motion.

Q21. What is the advantage and disadvantage of Fones technique?

Answer

Advantages: It is popular because it is very easy to learn.

Disadvantage: Rolled-gingival margins prevent removal of plaque from sulcus area.

Q22. What is scrub technique?

Answer

Scrub Technique

1. It is the simplest method.
2. Consists of merely placing the bristles next to the teeth and moving them 'back and forth' or scrubbing.

Advantage: It is easy to master.

Disadvantage: Poor plaque removal causes cervical abrasion and gingival recession.

Q23. What are the various types of motions used in powered toothbrush?

Answer

Powered Toothbrushes

They were introduced in 1939. Various types of motions used in powered toothbrushes are:
1. Reciprocal or 'back and forth'.
2. Circular.
3. Elliptical or combination.

Q24. When powered toothbrushes are recommended?

Answer

Powered toothbrushes are recommended for:
1. Individuals lacking fine motor skills.
2. Small children or handicapped or hospitalized patients who need to have their teeth cleaned by someone else.
3. Patients with orthodontic appliances.
4. Patients who prefer them.

Q25. What is the composition of toothpaste/dentifrice?

Answer

Composition of toothpaste:
1. Abrasives such as 20%–40% $CaCO_3$, $Ca_3(PO_4)_2$ both of which react with fluoride. Now, silicon oxides (SiO_2), aluminum oxide (Al_2O_3), granular polyvinyl chloride are used.
2. Humectants: 20%–40%; maintains moisture, e.g. glycerine, sorbitol, mannitol, propylene glycol.
3. Preservatives: Such as benzoic acid.
4. Thickening agents: Synthetic sodium carboxymethyl cellulose is used.
5. Water: 20%–40%.
6. Foaming agents: 1%–2% soap/detergent, e.g. sodium lauryl sulfate.
7. Flavoring and sweetening agents:
   a. Synthetic flavors and 2% essential oils, e.g. mint and others.
   b. Sweetening agents such as saccharin, sorbitol, mannitol.
8. Desensitizing agents: Up to 2% strontium salts, sodium fluoride, formalin, potassium nitrate and others.
9. Coloring and preservatives: Less than 1%.
10. Anticaries agents: Sodium monofluorophosphate, sodium fluoride and formalin.

Q26. What are the factors determining the selection of interdental aids?

Answer

Factors determining the selection of interdental aids are the type of embrasures:
1. *Type 1:* The interdental papilla fills up the embrasure. Dental floss is advised.
2. *Type 2:* Moderate papillary recession is seen in such situations, miniature interdental brushes and wood tips are recommended.
3. *Type 3:* Where there is complete loss of papilla and interdental gingiva is tightly bound to underlying bone (seen in diastema). Unitufted brushes are recommended.

Q27. What are the different types of dental floss?

Answer

1. Twisted or non-twisted.
2. Bonded or non-bonded.
3. Waxed or unwaxed.
4. Thick or thin.

Q28. What are the factors determining the choice of dental floss?

Answer

1. Tightness of tooth contacts.
2. Roughness of proximal surfaces.
3. The patient's manual dexterity.

Q29. What are interdental brushes?

Answer

Interdental brushes: They are cone-shaped or cylindrical brushes made of bristles mounted on a handle. Two types are available as given below:
1. Single-tufted brushes.
2. Small conical brushes: They are mainly useful to clean large, irregular concave tooth surfaces adjacent to wide interdental spaces.

Q30. What are wooden tips? How they are used?

Answer

Wooden tips are either with or without handle. Soft triangular wooden toothpicks such as Stim-U-Dent are placed in the interdental space in such a way that the base of the triangle rests on the gingiva and the sides are in contact with the proximal tooth surfaces and it is moved in and out of the embrasure removing soft deposits from the teeth and also mechanically stimulating the papillary gingiva, but its usefulness is limited to the facial surfaces in the anterior region of the mouth. Wooden toothpicks can be attached to a handle. For example, Perio-Aid and can be used on the facial and lingual surfaces throughout the mouth.

Q31. What are the functions of oral irrigator devices?

Answer

Oral irrigators clean non-adherent bacteria and debris from the oral cavity. It has been shown to disrupt and detoxify subgingival plaque and can be useful in delivering antimicrobial agents into periodontal pockets (subgingival irrigation).

Q32. What are the two types of irrigator tips for subgingival irrigation?

Answer

Currently, there are two types of irrigator tips useful for subgingival irrigation. One is the cannula type tip recommended for office use and other is a soft rubber tip for patient's use at home.

Q33. What are the ideal properties of a mouthwash?

Answer

Ideal Properties of a Mouthwash

1. Eliminate pathogenic microorganisms only.
2. Prevent development of resistant bacteria.
3. Exhibit substantivity.
4. Be safe to oral tissues at the recommended concentration.
5. Significantly reduce plaque formation and gingivitis.
6. Inhibit calcification of plaque to calculus.
7. Not stain and alter taste.
8. Not have adverse effects on teeth or dental materials.
9. Be easy to use.
10. Be inexpensive.

Q34. Classify antimicrobial agents.

Answer

Classification of Antimicrobial Agents

Depending on antimicrobial efficacy and substantivity.
1. First generation agent: Reduces plaque scores by 20%–50%, efficacy is limited by their poor retention in the oral cavity. Hence, used 4–6 times daily (poor substantivity). For examples, antibiotics, quaternary ammonium compounds, phenols and sanguinarine.
2. Second generation agents: These are retained longer in the oral cavity or tissues and slow release property provides overall reduction in plaque score by 70%–90% used 1–2 times daily (higher substantivity). For example, bisbiguanides.
3. Third generation agents: It should be effective against specific periodontopathic organisms. Yet to be developed clinically.

Q35. What is Addy's classification for chemicals used for supragingival plaque control?

Answer

1. Antibiotics: Penicillin, vancomycin, kanamycin, erythromycin, spiramycin, metronidazole.
2. Enzymes: Mucinase, protease, lipase, amylase, elastase, lactoperoxidase.
3. Quaternary ammonium compounds: Cetylpyridinium chloride, benzethonium chloride. benzalkonium chloride, domiphen bromide.
4. Bisbiguanides: Chlorhexidine, alexidine, octenidine/bispyridines.
5. Metallic salts: Copper, tin, zinc.
6. Herbal extracts: Sanguinarine.
7. Fluorides: Strontium fluoride.

8. Oxygenating agents: Hydrogen peroxide.
9. Phenolic compounds: Thymol, menthol, eucalyptol.
10. Other antiseptics: Iodine, povidone iodine, sodium hypochlorite.

Q36. What are the indications of chlorhexidine as a mouthwash?

Answer

Indications and Uses

1. Used as an adjunct to mechanical oral hygiene in initial periodontal therapy.
2. During postsurgical period.
3. Improves healing after routine oral surgical procedures and in the postoperative management of immediate denture construction.
4. Patients wearing fixed orthodontic appliances or intermaxillary fixation devices will benefit from a daily rinse with a 0.2% chlorhexidine solution (also available in 0.12% concentration).
5. For handicapped patients whose plaque control and gingival status are often very poor.
6. Chlorhexidine will help to control plaque accumulation in patients with drug-induced gingival overgrowth.
7. In medically compromised patients who suffer from recurrent generalized oral infections.
8. It can also be advised in patients with local, oral infections such as denture-induced stomatitis, aphthous ulceration, dry socket and acute ulcerative gingivitis.
9. Finally, it can be used as a prophylactic rinse in the prevention of postextraction bacteremia, dry sockets and to reduce the bacterial content of the aerosol sprays during the ultrasonic scaling.

Q37. What are the disadvantages/unwanted effects of chlorhexidine?

Answer

Disadvantages/unwanted effects are as follows:
1. Extrinsic staining of teeth, i.e. brown stains.
2. Painful, desquamative lesions on the oral mucosa may be associated with burning sensation.
3. Impaired taste sensation.
4. Parotid swelling is rare: Due to mechanical obstruction of parotid duct.
5. Dryness and soreness of mucosa.

Q38. What is the mechanism of action of chlorhexidine?

Answer

It has a broad spectrum of antibacterial activity. In general, gram-positive bacteria are more susceptible as compared to gram-negative bacteria. In relatively high concentrations, chlorhexidine is bactericidal, but low concentrations may be bacteriostatic to susceptible bacteria. The cationic molecules of chlorhexidine bind readily to the oppositely charged cell wall and interfere with the membrane transport initiating a leakage of low molecular weight substances. In high concentrations, chlorhexidine penetrates the cell and causes precipitation of the cytoplasm. This explains the bactericidal action of bisbiguanides in general.

Q39. What are the two concentrations in which chlorhexidine is commercially available?

Answer

Commercially, available products in the concentration of 0.2% are Rexidine, Hexidine, Clohex, in 0.12%, as PerioGard.

Q40. What is pincushion effect?

Answer

It could be explained as follows: One charged end of chlorhexidine (dicationic) molecule binds to the tooth surface whereas the other remains available to initiate the interaction with the bacterial membrane as the microorganism approaches the tooth surface is called 'pincushion effect'.

Q41. What is composition of essential oil rinse?

Answer

Essential Oil Rinse

The rinse contains thymol, eucalyptol, menthol and methylsalicylate. It has been proved to be effective in reducing plaque and gingival scores. Commercially available as Listerine®.

Q42. What are the advantages of disclosing agents?

Answer

Disclosing agents offers the following advantages:
1. Discloses plaque.
2. Permits patients to evaluate their performance at home.

Q43. What are the various disclosing agents?

Answer

1. Erythrosine dye: FDC No. 3.
2. Two-tone dye:
   a. FDC No. 3: Red.
   b. No. 3: Green.
      It can differentiate older to newer plaque; old plaque stains deep violet and new plaque pale violet.
3. Plak-lite system: Available as wafers/tablets or solutions, which are swished around the mouth and excess dye is removed by rinsing the mouth.

CHAPTER 41

Principles of Periodontal Surgery

Q1. What are the indications of periodontal surgery?

Answer
1. Areas with irregular bony contours, deep craters and others requiring a surgical approach.
2. Deep pockets where complete removal of root irritants is not possible, especially in inaccessible areas like molars and premolar areas.
3. In cases of grade II and III furcation involvement, where apart from removing local irritants, necessary root resection or hemisection can be considered.
4. Infrabony pockets in non-accessible areas, which are non-responsive toward non-surgical methods.
5. Persistent inflammation in areas with moderate and deep pockets.
6. Correction of mucogingival problems.

Q2. What are the contraindications of periodontal surgery?

Answer
These may be oral or systemic:
1. In patients of advanced age where teeth may last for life without resorting to radical treatment (procedures indicated in a person of 60 years of age may not be justified in someone of 70 years of age).
2. Patients with systemic diseases such as cardiovascular disease, malignancy, liver diseases, blood disorders, uncontrolled-diabetes, consultation with the patient's physician is essential.
3. Where thorough subgingival scaling and good home care will resolve or control the lesion.
4. Where patient motivation is inadequate.
5. In the presence of infection.
6. Where the prognosis is so poor that tooth loss is inevitable.

Q3. What are the general principles of surgery?

Answer
1. Preparation of the patient.
2. The general conditions that is common to all periodontal surgical techniques.
3. Complications that may occur during or after surgery.

Q4. What are the general conditions that are common to all patients?

Answer
The following are the general conditions that are common to all patients:
1. Premedication.
2. Sedation and anesthesia.
3. Tissue management.
4. Suturing.

Q5. Describe premedication.

Answer
For normal patients their use is not clearly demonstrated. The prophylactic use of antibiotics has been advocated for both medically compromised patients as well as patients undergoing bone-grafting procedures. Emergency equipment should be readily available at all the times. All the measures should be taken to prevent the transmission of infections. These include the use of disposable gloves, surgical masks and protective eyewear. All surfaces that may be contaminated with blood or saliva and cannot be sterilized, must be covered with aluminum foil/plastic wrap. Ultrasonic scaling is contraindicated in patients with infectious diseases, as it generates aerosols and special care should be taken while using it (preprocedural mouthrinsing).

Q6. Classify suturing materials.

Answer

Suturing materials are classified as either non-absorbable or absorbable:
1. Non-absorbable:
   a. Natural: For example, braided-silk.
   b. Synthetic: For example, Dacron-coated and impregnated with Teflon.
2. Absorbable:
   a. Natural: For example, surgical gut.
   b. Synthetic: For example, polyglycolic acid derivatives like Vicryl.

Q7. What are the goals of suturing?

Answer

1. Maintains hemostasis.
2. Permits healing by primary intention.
3. Reduces postoperative pain.
4. Permits proper flap position.
5. Prevents bone exposure resulting in delayed healing and unnecessary resorption.

Q8. What are the different suturing techniques?

Answer

Different suturing techniques are as follows:
1. Interrupted suture:
   a. Direct or loop suture.
   b. Figure eight suture.
   c. Horizontal mattress.
   d. Vertical mattress.
   e. Distal wedge or anchor suture.
   f. Periosteal suturing.
2. Continuous suture:
   a. Papillary sling.
   b. Horizontal mattress.
   c. Vertical mattress.

Q9. What are the different parts of surgical needles?

Answer

1. Eye.
2. Body: Widest point of the needle and is referred to as the 'grasping area'.
3. Point: Point of the tip can be conventional or reverse cutting.

Q10. Describe how to manage the tissues during surgery.

Answer

Tissue Management

1. *Operate gently and carefully:* In addition to being most considerate to the patient, tissue manipulation should be gentle because it produces excessive tissue injury; causes postoperative discomfort and delays healing.
2. Observe the patient at all times.
3. *Be certain the instruments are sharp:* Dull instruments will cause unnecessary trauma, because of excess force usually applied to compensate for their ineffectiveness.

CHAPTER 42

Gingival Curettage

Q1. Define gingival curettage. What are its types?

Answer

The term curettage is used in periodontics to mean the scraping of gingival wall of a periodontal pocket to separate diseased soft tissue.

Types

1. *Gingival curettage:* Consists of removal of inflamed soft tissue lateral to pocket wall:
   a. *Subgingival curettage:* It is a procedure that is performed apical to epithelial attachment.
   b. *Inadvertent curettage:* Curettage that is done unintentionally during scaling and root planing.
2. Surgical curettage, chemical curettage, ultrasonic curettage.

Q2. What is rationale of gingival curettage?

Answer

The main accomplishment of curettage is the removal of chronically inflamed granulation tissue that forms in the lateral wall of the periodontal pocket.

Q3. What are the indications of curettage?

Answer

1. Can be performed as a part of new attachment in moderately deep infrabony pockets located in accessible areas where a type of 'closed surgery' is advised.
2. Can be done as a non-definite procedure to reduce inflammation prior to pocket elimination procedures like flap surgeries.
3. It can also be performed in patients where extensive surgical procedures are contraindicated like aging, systemic complications, etc. where the treatment is compromised and prognosis is impaired.
4. Curettage is frequently performed on recall visits as a method of maintenance treatment for areas of recurrent inflammation and pocket depth, particularly where pocket reduction surgery has previously been performed.

Q4. What are the various techniques used to accomplish gingival curettage?

Answer

Basic Technique

1. After adequate local anesthesia, the correct curette is selected and adapted in such a way that the cutting edge is against the tissues. The instrument is inserted so as to engage the inner lining of the pocket wall and is carried along the soft tissue wall usually in a horizontal stroke.
2. In subgingival curettage, the tissue attached between the bottom of pocket and the alveolar crest is removed with a scooping motion of the curette to the tooth surface. The area is flushed to remove debris.
3. Other techniques include ENAP, caustic drugs and ultrasonic curettage.

Q5. What is excisional new attachment procedure (ENAP)?

Answer

It is a definitive subgingival curettage procedure performed with a knife. It was developed by United States Naval Corps. The technique is:

1. After adequate local anesthesia, an internal bevel incision is made from margin of free gingiva apically below the base of pocket; it is carried all around the tooth surface, attempting to retain as much interdental tissue as possible.
2. The excised tissue is then removed with a curette and the root surface is planed to a smooth hard consistency.

3. Approximate wound edges if necessary, place sutures and a periodontal dressing.

Q6. What are different caustic drugs used for curettage?

Answer

Caustic Drugs

Drugs such as sodium sulfide, antiformin and phenol have been used to induce chemical curettage of the lateral wall of the pocket. Disadvantage is the extent of tissue destruction with these drugs cannot be controlled.

CHAPTER 43

Gingivectomy

Q1. Define gingivectomy and gingivoplasty.
Answer
1. Gingivectomy is the excision of the soft tissue wall of the pocket (its objective is the elimination of pockets).
2. Gingivoplasty is the recontouring of gingiva that has lost its physiologic form rather than elimination of pockets.

Q2. What are the prerequisites of gingivectomy?
Answer
The basic prerequisites for gingivectomy are as follows:
1. There should be adequate zone of attached gingiva, so that excision of part of it will still leave a functionally adequate zone.
2. The underlying alveolar bone must be in normal or nearly normal form. If there is bone loss it should be of horizontal in nature.
3. There should be no infrabony defects or pockets.

Q3. What are the indications of gingivectomy?
Answer
1. Eliminate supra-alveolar pockets and abscesses.
2. Remove fibrous or edematous enlargements of the gingiva.
3. Transform rolled or blunted margins to physiologic form.
4. Create more esthetic form in cases in which exposure of the anatomic crown has not fully occurred.
5. Create bilateral symmetry (where the gingival margin of one incisor has receded somewhat more than that of the adjacent incisor).
6. Expose additional clinical crown to gain added retention for restorative procedures (access to subgingival areas, etc.).
7. Correct gingival craters.

Q4. What are the contraindications for gingivectomy and gingivoplasty?
Answer
Gingivectomy and gingivoplasty are not indicated in the following situations:
1. In the presence of thick alveolar edges, interdental craters or bizarre crestal bone form.
2. When infrabony pockets are present.
3. If pockets extends till/below the mucogingival junction.
4. Inadequate oral hygiene maintenance by the patients.
5. Uncooperative patients.
6. Medically compromised patients.
7. Dentinal hypersensitivity before the surgical procedure (requires considerable preparation of the patient mentally and is not exactly a contraindication).
8. Esthetically challenging areas, especially in the maxillary anterior region.

Q5. What are the types of gingivectomy?
Answer
1. Surgical gingivectomy.
2. Gingivectomy by electrosurgery.
3. Laser gingivectomy.
4. Gingivectomy by chemosurgery.

Q6. What are the incisions used for surgical gingivectomy?
Answer
The incision is started apical to the points marking the course of the pockets and is directed coronally to a point between the base of the pocket and the crest of the bone. Discontinuous or continuous incisions may be used. The incision should be beveled at approximately 45 degrees to the tooth surface and should recreate as far as possible the normal festooned pattern of gingival.

Q7. What is the frequency and classes of electrodes used for electrosurgery?

Answer

It uses high frequency current of 1.5–7.5 million cycles per second.

There are three classes of electrodes used:
1. Single wire electrodes for incising and excising.
2. Loop electrodes for planing tissues.
3. Heavy bulkier electrodes for coagulation procedures.

Q8. What are the four types of electrosurgical techniques available?

Answer

The four types of electrosurgical techniques, which are available are as follows:
1. *Electrosection:* Three procedures are performed such as incising, excising and planing.
2. *Electrocoagulation:* Used to prevent hemorrhage.
3. *Electrofulguration:* Uses high voltage current. It has limited application in dentistry.
4. *Electrodesiccation:* Uses dehydrating current and least used, as it is a dangerous technique.

Q9. What are the advantages and disadvantages of gingivectomy by electrosurgery?

Answer

Advantages

Permits adequate contouring of the tissues and controls hemorrhage.

Disadvantages

1. Cannot be used in patients with poorly shielded cardiac pacemaker.
2. Causes unpleasant odor.
3. If it touches the bone irreparable damage may result.
4. Heat generated by this may cause tissue damage and areas of cemental necrosis.

Q10. What are the indications of electrosurgery?

Answer

1. Removal of gingival enlargements.
2. Gingivoplasty.
3. Relocation of frenum and muscle attachments.
4. Incision of periodontal abscesses and pericoronal abscess.

Q11. What are the electrosurgical techniques used for various periodontal procedures?

Answer

1. *For gingivoplasty:* Needle electrodes and diamond-shaped electrodes are used for festooning. In all reshaping procedures, electrodes are activated and moved in a concise 'shaving' motion (cutting and coagulating current is used).
2. *For abscess drainage:* Incisions can be made with the needle electrode.
3. *For hemostasis:* Ball electrode is used.
4. *For relocation of frenum and muscle attachment:* Loop electrode is used.

Q12. What are the most commonly used lasers for gingivectomy?

Answer

The most commonly used lasers are carbon dioxide and neodymium-doped yttrium aluminum garnet (Nd:YAG) lasers. They are used for excision of gingival over growth.

Q13. What are the chemicals used for gingivectomy?

Answer

The chemicals used are 5% paraformaldehyde or potassium hydroxide to remove gingiva.

Q14. What are the disadvantages of chemosurgery?

Answer

1. Their depth of action cannot be controlled, hence it may also injure normal tissues.
2. Gingival remodeling is not possible.
3. Healing is delayed.

CHAPTER 44

Periodontal Flap

Q1. Define periodontal surgery.

Answer

Periodontal surgery (open) is defined as intentional severing or incising of gingival tissue with the purpose of controlling or eliminating periodontal disease.

Q2. Define periodontal flap.

Answer

A periodontal flap is a section of gingiva and/or mucosa, surgically elevated from the underlying tissues to provide visibility of and access to the bone and root surface.

Q3. What are the indications for a flap surgery?

Answer

1. Gain access for root debridement.
2. Reduction or elimination of pocket depth, so that patient can maintain the root surfaces free of plaque.
3. Reshaping soft and hard tissues to attain a harmonious topography (physiologic architecture).
4. Regeneration of alveolar bone, periodontal ligament and cementum.

Q4. Classify periodontal flaps.

Answer

According to Thickness of the Flap/Bone Exposure after Flap Reflection

Full thickness/mucoperiosteal flap: All the soft tissues including the periosteum are elevated.

Partial thickness/mucosal flap/split thickness flap: Reflection of only the epithelium and a layer of underlying connective tissue, the bone is covered by a layer of connective tissue including periosteum.

According to the Placement of the Flap after Surgery

Non-displaced flap: The flap is returned and sutured back in its original position.

Displaced flaps: The flap is repositioned coronal, apical or lateral to its original position. However, palatal flaps cannot be displaced due to the absence of unattached gingiva.

According to Design of the Flap/Management of the Papilla

Conventional flaps: Splitting the papilla into a facial half and lingual/palatal half. For example, modified Widman flap, undisplaced flap, apically displaced flap.

Papilla preservation flaps: Entire papilla is incorporated into one of the flaps.

Q5. What are the indications for a full thickness and a partial thickness flap?

Answer

Full thickness: If osseous surgery is contemplated.

Partial thickness: For displacing flaps in the presence of dehiscence and fenestrations.

Q6. What are the indications for conventional flaps?

Answer

1. When the interdental areas are too narrow to permit the preservation of flap.
2. When there is a need for displacing flaps.

Q7. What are the indications for a papilla preservation flap?

Answer

1. Where esthetics is of concern.
2. Where bone regeneration techniques are attempted.

Q8. What are the incisions given for a conventional flap?

Answer

1. Horizontal incision:
   - Internal bevel incision
   - Crevicular incision
   - Interdental incision.
2. Vertical incision:
   - Oblique releasing incision.

Q9. What type of incision is given for a papilla preservation flap?

Answer

Crevicular incision with no incisions across the interdental papilla is given.

Q10. What is internal bevel incision?

Answer

An internal bevel incision starts at a distance (1–2 mm) from the gingival margin and is aimed at the bone crest. It is a basic incision to most of the flap procedures. It is also known as first incision, reverse bevel incision. No. 15 and No. 11 surgical scalpels are most commonly used.

Q11. What are the objectives of an internal bevel incision?

Answer

It accomplishes three important objectives:
1. Removes pocket lining.
2. Conserves relatively uninvolved outer surface of the gingiva.
3. It produces a sharp, thin flap margin for adaptation to tooth—bone junction.

Q12. What is crevicular incision?

Answer

It is also termed as the second incision, is made from the base of the pocket to the crest of the bone. The incision is carried around the entire tooth. No. 12B blade is used. This results in V-shaped wedge of tissue containing inflamed granulomatous tissue consisting of lateral wall of the pocket, junctional epithelium and connective tissue fibers between the base of the pocket and crest of the bone.

Q13. What is interdental incision?

Answer

After the crevicular incision is given, a periosteal elevator is used to separate the flap from the bone. With this access, the surgeon is able to make the third or interdental incision, to separate the collar of the gingiva that is left around the tooth. The Orban knife is usually utilized for this incision. A curette or a large scaler (U15/30) can be used to remove the gingiva around the tooth.

Q14. What is envelope flap?

Answer

A flap with no vertical incision is known as envelope flap. This flap is reflected using only horizontal incision.

Q15. When and how to perform vertical incision?

Answer

It can be done on one or both the ends of the horizontal incision. If the flap has to be displaced the incisions at both ends should be made. Vertical incisions should be made extending beyond mucogingival junction for easy displacement of flap. Another indication for vertical incision is in the presence of isolated deep pockets.

Q16. Name the areas where vertical incisions are avoided.

Answer

In general, vertical incisions are avoided:
1. In lingual or palatal areas.
2. At the center of the interdental papilla or over the radicular surface.

Q17. Where are the vertical incisions made?

Answer

They are made along the line angles of the tooth, avoid short flaps with long, apically directed incisions as it compromises blood supply to the flap.

Q18. What are the flap techniques for pocket therapy?

Answer

The periodontal flap is one of the most frequently employed procedure particularly for eliminating/reducing moderate to deep pockets in posterior areas. There are three flap techniques available in current use. They are:
1. Modified Widman flap.
2. Undisplaced flap.
3. Apically displaced flap.

Q19. Who devised modified Widman flap?

Answer

Modified Widman flap was devised by Ramfjord and Nissle in 1974.

CHAPTER 44 Periodontal Flap

Q20. What are the techniques in the variation of palatal flap?

Answer

1. Usual internal bevel incision, followed by crevicular and interdental incisions, but if the tissue is thick horizontal gingivectomy incision is made, followed by an internal bevel incision. Thinning of the flap should be done prior to reflection of the flap.
2. The apical portion of the scalloping incision should be narrower than the line angle area, because the palatal root tapers apically, rounded scallop will result in improper adaptation of the flap around root.

Q21. Which flap technique is also called internal bevel gingivectomy?

Answer

The undisplaced flap is otherwise called internal bevel gingivectomy, since the soft tissue pocket wall is removed with the initial incision.

Q22. What are the indications of apically displaced flap?

Answer

1. Improves accessibility.
2. It also eliminates the pocket by transforming the previously unattached keratinized pocket wall into attached tissues (offers dual function).

Q23. Which flap technique is most suitable for regenerative therapy?

Answer

1. Papilla preservation.
2. Conventional flap with only crevicular incision.

Q24. What are the indications of distal molar surgery?

Answer

To treat periodontal pockets on the distal surface of a terminal tooth.

Q25. What are the indications for sulcular or crevicular incision?

Answer

1. In the presence of narrow band of keratinized gingiva.
2. In moderate periodontal pockets especially in the esthetic zone.
3. Is indicated whenever osseous surgery is contemplated (e.g. bone grafts, guided tissue regeneration, etc.).
4. As a basic horizontal incision in any type of flap surgery.

Q26. Name the various designs in distal molar surgery.

Answer

1. Triangular.
2. Square.
3. Parallel.
4. H design.

Q27. Compare flap procedure with gingivectomy.

Answer

Comparison between flap procedure and gingivectomy		
Features	Flap	Gingivectomy
Reattachment	Possible	Not possible
Healing	Primary	Secondary
Bleeding	Low	High
Preservation of keratinized tissue	Yes	No
Treatment of osseous defects	Possible	Not possible

CHAPTER 45

Osseous Surgery

Q1. What is the AAP definition of osseous surgery?
Answer

According to the American Academy of Periodontology (AAP); it is defined as "procedures to modify bone support altered by periodontal disease, either by reshaping the alveolar process to achieve physiologic form, without the removal of the alveolar supporting bone or by the removal of some alveolar bone, thus changing the position of crestal bone relative to the tooth root."

Q2. Define osteoplasty according to AAP.
Answer

Osteoplasty is defined as reshaping of the alveolar process to achieve a more physiologic form without removal of supporting bones.

Q3. Define ostectomy according to AAP.
Answer

Ostectomy is defined as the excision of bone or portion of a bone in periodontics, it is done to correct or reduce deformities caused by periodontitis and includes removal of the supporting bone.

Q4. What are the types of osseous surgery?
Answer

Depending on the relative position of the interdental bone to radicular bone, osseous surgery is of following types:
1. *Positive architecture:* When the radicular bone is apical to the interdental bone.
2. *Negative architecture:* If the interdental bone is more apical than the radicular bone.
3. *Flat architecture:* It is the reduction of interdental bone to the same height as radicular bone.
4. *Ideal:* When the bone is consistently more coronal on the interproximal surface than on the facial and lingual surfaces.

Depending on the thoroughness of the osseous reshaping techniques, osseous surgery is of following types:

1. *Definitive osseous reshaping:* Implies that further reshaping would not improve the overall result.
2. *Compromise osseous reshaping:* It indicates a bone pattern that cannot be improved without significant osseous removal, which would be detrimental to the overall result.

Osseous surgery can also be:
1. *Additive:* Directed toward restoring the bone to original levels.
2. *Subtractive:* It is designed to restore the form of the pre-existing alveolar bone to the level existing at the time of surgery or slightly apical to this level.

Q5. What are the indications of osseous resective surgery?
Answer

1. One-walled angular defects.
2. Thick, bony margins.
3. Shallow crater formations.

Q6. What are the contraindications of resective osseous surgery?
Answer

1. Anatomic factors such as close proximity of the roots to the maxillary antrum or the ramus.
2. Age.
3. Systemic health.
4. Improper oral hygiene.
5. High caries index.
6. Extreme root sensitivity.
7. Advanced periodontitis.
8. Unacceptable esthetic result.

Q7. What are the examinations carried out prior to surgery?
Answer

Clinical examination and probing is carried out, which determines the presence and the depth of periodontal pockets and also gives a general sense of the bony topography. Transgingival probing or sounding under local anesthesia confirms the extent and configuration of the infrabony component or furcation defects.

Q8. Enumerate the hand instruments used for resective osseous surgery.

answer

Hand instruments include:
1. Rongeurs—Friedman and Blumenthal.
2. Interproximal files—Schluger and Sugarman.
3. Back action chisels.
4. Ochsenbein chisels.

Q9. Enumerate the rotary instruments used for osseous resective surgery.

Answer

Rotary instruments include:
1. Carbide round burs.
2. Slow-speed handpiece.
3. Diamond burs.

Q10. What are the steps in osseous resective surgery?

Answer

1. Vertical grooving.
2. Radicular blending.
3. Flattening of interproximal bone.
4. Gradualizing marginal bone.

Q11. What is vertical grooving?

Answer

It is performed to reduce the thickness of alveolar housing and it provides continuity from the interproximal surface into the radicular surface. It is the first step of the resective process and is usually performed with rotary instruments such as round, carbide or diamond burs.

Q12. When is vertical grooving indicated?

Answer

Vertical grooving is indicated in thick bony margins, shallow crater formation.

Q13. What are the contraindications for vertical grooving?

Answer

Vertical grooving is contraindicated in areas with close root proximity or thin alveolar housing.

Q14. What is radicular blending?

Answer

It is the second step of the osseous reshaping technique. It is the continuation of the first step and it attempts to gradualize the bone over the entire radicular surface and thereby provides a smooth, blended surface for good flap adaptation.

Q15. What are the indications of radicular blending?

Answer

1. Thick bony margins, shallow crater formation.
2. Grade-I and grade-II furcation involvements.

Q16. What is flattening of the interproximal bone?

Answer

It requires removal of very small amount of supporting bone. This step is also best-utilized in areas where there are combined defects, i.e. coronally one-walled defect and apically three-walled defect, so that it is helpful in obtaining good flap closure and hence improved healing.

Q17. When is the flattening of the interproximal bone indicated?

Answer

It is indicated when interproximal bone levels vary horizontally, e.g. one wall defects or hemiseptal defects.

Q18. When is flattening of interproximal bone contraindicated?

Answer

It cannot be utilized in advanced defects, where removal of inordinate amounts of bone may be required.

Q19. What is gradualizing marginal bone?

Answer

The final step in the osseous resective technique is also an ostectomy procedure. Bone removal is minimal, but necessary to provide a sound regular base for the gingival tissue to follow. Failure to do so may result in 'widow's peaks'.

Q20. What are widow's peaks?

Answer

Schluger in 1949, described widow's peak as the residual pieces of cortical bone left over facial or lingual line angle from the horizontal grooving that form a crater in a mesiodistal direction.

Q21. What is spheroiding/parabolizing and scribing?

Answer

Spheroiding/parabolizing: It is the removal of supporting bone to produce a positive gingival and osseous architecture.

Scribing: It is a technique by which a high speed rotary instrumentation is used to outline on the radicular bone, the bone, which is to be removed by hand instrumentation.

Q22. What are the possible outcomes of surgical periodontal therapy?

Answer

1. New attachment.
2. Long junctional epithelium.
3. Root resorption/ankylosis.
4. Recurrence of pocket.

Q23. Enumerate the methods to evaluate new attachment and bone regeneration.

Answer

1. Clinical method.
2. Radiographic method.
3. Surgical re-entry.
4. Histological method.

Q24. What are the clinical methods to evaluate the new attachment and bone regeneration?

Answer

1. Probing depth measurements (pre- and post-treatment).
2. Clinical gingival indices.
3. Determination of attachment level.

Q25. What are the drawbacks of radiographic methods?

Answer

1. Standardized techniques for reproducible positioning of the film and tubing are very difficult.
2. The radiograph may not show the entire topography of the area before or after the treatment.
3. Thin bony trabeculae, which was present before treatment may go undetected because minimal amount of mineralized tissue must be present to be seen or registered on the radiograph.

Q26. What is surgical re-entry?

Answer

This can give the best view of the state of the bone crest that can be compared with the one taken during the initial surgical intervention and can also be subjected to measurements. Even models can be used to appreciate the results of the therapy (pre- and post-treatment).

Q27. What are the shortcomings of surgical re-entry method?

Answer

1. It requires a frequently unnecessary second operation.
2. It does not show the type of attachment that exists (epithelial or connective tissue attachments).

Q28. What is the histological method of evaluation of new attachment and bone regeneration?

Answer

The type of attachment can only be determined by the histological analysis of the tissue block taken from the healed area.

Q29. Enumerate the reconstructive surgical procedures.

Answer

The following reconstructive surgical techniques have been proposed:
1. Non-graft-associated new attachment.
2. Graft-associated new attachment.
3. Combination of both.

Q30. What are the conditions in which new attachment can be achieved without the use of grafts?

Answer

New attachment can be achieved without the use of grafts in:
1. Meticulously treated three-walled defects (infrabony defect).
2. Perioendodontal abscesses.
3. When the destructive procedure has occurred very rapidly. For example, after treatment of pockets, which had acute periodontal abscess.

Q31. What are the various techniques of non-graft-associated new attachment?

Answer

1. Removal of junctional and pocket epithelium.
2. Prevention of epithelial migration.
3. Guided tissue regeneration (GTR).
4. Clot stabilization, wound protection and space creation.
5. Preparation of the root surface (root biomodification).

Q32. What are the methods used in the removal of junctional and pocket epithelium?

Answer

1. *Curettage:* Only 50% of junctional epithelium and pocket epithelium can be removed.
2. *Chemical agents:* Mostly used in conjunction with curettage. The most commonly used drugs are sodium sulfide, phenol, camphor, sodium hypochlorite and antiformin. The main disadvantage is that the depth of action cannot be controlled.
3. *Ultrasonic methods:* It is again not very useful, because of lack of clinician's tactile sense, while using these methods.

4. *Surgical methods:* It include:
   - Excisional new attachment procedure with internal bevel incision (ENAP)
   - Gingivectomy procedure
   - Modified Widman flap
   - Coronal displacement of the flap.

Q33. What is guided tissue regeneration (GTR)?

Answer

This concept is based on the assumption that periodontal ligament cells have the potential for regeneration of the attachment apparatus of the tooth.

Q34. What are the two types of membranes used in GTR?

Answer

Two types of membranes have been used.

Degradable: Collagen, polylactic acid, Vicryl (polyglactin 910) and Guidor membrane.

Non-degradable: They must be removed in three to six weeks time, e.g. Millipore, Teflon membrane, Gore-Tex periodontal material.

Q35. What are the substances used for root biomodification?

Answer

Substances used to condition the root surface, for attachment of new connective, tissue fibers. These include citric acid, fibronectin and tetracycline.

Q36. Who reported the actions of citric acid?

Answer

The actions of citric acid have been reported by Register and Burdick in 1975.

Q37. What is the role of citric acid in root biomodification?

Answer

When used with pH 1.0 for 2–3 minutes on root surface, after surgical debridement, it produces a surface demineralization, which in turn induces cementogenesis and attachment of collagen fibers. The following are the actions of citric acid:
1. It removes the smear layer and may open dentinal tubules, thus allowing cementum to form within these tubules creating the blunderbuss effect and produce cementum pins. This could be associated with accelerated cementogenesis.
2. It has also been shown to expose collagen fibers on the root surface, which may splice with the collagen fibers of a soft tissue graft or flap (called collagen splicing) resulting in collagen adhesion without cementum formation and accelerated healing.
3. Epithelium does not migrate apically because of the accelerated healing either by connective tissue attachment or a collagen adhesion may occur before epithelium migrates.
4. Finally, citric acid may demineralize small bits of residual calculus, disinfect the root surface and aid in removing endotoxins.

Q38. What are growth factors? Name a few.

Answer

They are polypeptide molecules released by the cells in the inflamed area that regulates events in wound healing. These factors are primarily secreted by macrophages, endothelial cells, fibroblasts and platelets. They include:
- Platelet-derived growth factor (PDGF)
- Insulin-like growth factor (IGF)
- Fibroblast growth factor (FGF)
- Transforming growth factor-alpha and -beta (TGF-α and -β).

Q39. What are the roles of growth factors?

Answer

Growth factors can be used to control events during periodontal wound healing, e.g. promoting proliferation of fibroblasts from periodontal ligament thereby favoring bone formation.

Q40. What are enamel matrix proteins?

Answer

These are based on the observations that amelogenin secreted by Hertwig's epithelial root sheath during tooth development can induce acellular cementum formation, which is believed to favor periodontal regeneration, e.g. Emdogain approved by Food and Drug Administration (FDA).

Q41. What are bone morphogenetic proteins (BMPs)?

Answer

Bone morphogenetic proteins are a form of unique group of proteins with the transforming growth factor-beta (TGF-β) superfamily of genes and have pivotal roles in regulation of:
- Bone induction
- Maintenance
- Repair.

Q42. What is a graft?

Answer

Graft is a viable tissue/organ that after removal from donor site is implanted/transplanted within the host tissue, which is then repaired, restored and remodeled.

Q43. What is xenograft or heterograft?
Answer

The donor of the graft is from a species different from the host.

Q44. What is allograft or homograft?
Answer

A tissue transfer between individuals of the same species, but with non-identical genes.

Q45. What is an autograft?
Answer

A tissue transfer from one position to a new position in the same individual.

Q46. What is an alloplast?
Answer

A graft of inert synthetic material, which is sometimes called implant material.

Q47. What is osteoinduction?
Answer

A process by which the graft material is capable of promoting cementogenesis, osteogenesis and new periodontal ligament.

Q48. What is osteoconduction?
Answer

The graft material acts as a passive matrix, like a trellis or scaffolding for new bone to cover.

Q49. What is contact inhibition?
Answer

The process by which the graft material prevents apical proliferation of the epithelium.

Q50. What are the ideal requirements of a bone graft material?
Answer

- Biologic acceptability
- Predictability
- Clinical feasibility
- Minimal postoperative hazards
- Minimal postoperative sequelae
- Good patient acceptance.

Q51. What is intraoral autograft?
Answer

It is the tissue transfer from one area to another in the same individual, sources of intraoral autografts include healing extraction wound, bone from edentulous ridges, immature bone removed during osteoplasty and osteotomy, bone removed from a predetermined site like tori and symphysis.

Q52. What is osseous coagulum?
Answer

Rationale of this technique is that small particles of donor bone are better resorbed and replaced than the larger particles. This technique uses small particles of donor bone and hence it provides additional surface area for the interaction of cellular and vascular elements. Sources of the implant material include the lingual ridge on the mandible, exostosis, tori, edentulous ridges and the bone distal to the terminal tooth.

Q53. What are the disadvantages of osseous coagulum?
Answer

1. Low predictability.
2. Inability to procure adequate material.
3. Inability to use aspiration for large defects, which lead to poor surgical visibility.

Q54. What is bone blend?
Answer

It uses an autoclaved plastic capsule and pestle. Bone is removed from the predetermined site with chisels or Rongeur forceps, placed in the capsule with a few drops of saline and triturated for 60 seconds to a workable plastic-like mass and is packed into the bony defect.

Q55. What are the sources of intraoral cancellous bone marrow chips?
Answer

Intraoral cancellous bone marrow chips can be obtained from:
1. *Maxillary tuberosity:* It contains good amount of cancellous bone with foci of red marrow and the bone is removed with a cutting Rongeur.
2. *Edentulous areas:* The bone is removed with curette.
3. *Healing sockets:* They are allowed to heal for 8–12 weeks and the apical portion is utilized as donor material.

Q56. What is bone swaging?
Answer

This technique requires presence of an edentulous area adjacent to the defect from which the bone is pushed into contact with root surface without fracturing the bone at its base.

Q57. What are the disadvantages of bone swaging?
Answer

1. It is technically difficult.
2. Its usefulness is limited.

Q58. What are the extra oral sources of bone grafts?
Answer

Iliac autograft/extraoral hip marrow: The use of iliac cancellous bone marrow has shown good results in bony defects with varying number of walls and furcation defects.

Q59. What are the disadvantages of iliac autografts?
Answer

1. Additional surgical trauma.
2. Postoperative morbidity infection, exfoliation, sequestration.
3. Root resorption.
4. Rapid recurrence of the defect.

Q60. What are the commercially available allografts?
Answer

Freeze-dried bone allograft (FDBA): It is an osteoconductive material, varying results have been observed using this material. Average bone fill of 50% has been reported.

Demineralized freeze-dried bone allograft (DFDBA): Demineralization process exposes the components of bone matrix termed as bone morphogenic protein, e.g. osteogenin, which is a bone inductive protein isolated from the extracellular matrix of human bones. Hence, this is an osteoinductive material.

Q61. Give some examples for xenografts.
Answer

Examples of xenograft are calf bone, kiel bone, anorganic bone.

Q62. What are the types of calcium phosphate ceramics?
Answer

Coral-derived materials: Two types of materials are available, natural coral and coral-derived porous hydroxyapatite (both are proven to be biocompatible).

Combined techniques: A combination of both graft and non-graft associated methods have been proposed, e.g. combination of barrier techniques with bone grafts have been suggested by many authors.

Q63. What is platelet-rich fibrin (PRF)?
Answer

Platelet-rich fibrin is a 2nd generation platelet concentrate. First developed by Choukroun et al in France. It is prepared from the patient's own blood sample. The blood sample is taken without anticoagulant in a 10 mL tube and immediately centrifuged at 3,000 rpm for 10 minutes and a fibrin clot is obtained. PRF helps in providing a high concentration of growth factors.

Platelet-derived growth factor (PDGF), insulin-like growth factor (IGF), transforming growth factor-beta (TGF-β) and cytokines at the site of wound healing. In this way PRF ensures faster healing and regeneration of periodontal tissues.

CHAPTER 46

Mucogingival Surgery

Q1. Define periodontal plastic surgery.

Answer

Periodontal plastic surgery is defined as "surgical procedures performed to correct or eliminate anatomic, developmental or traumatic deformities of the gingiva or alveolar mucosa."

Q2. What is mucogingival surgery?

Answer

According to Glickman, mucogingival surgery consists of "plastic surgical procedures for the correction of gingiva, mucous membrane relationships that complicate periodontal diseases and may interfere with the success of periodontal treatment."

Q3. What are mucogingival problems?

Answer

Mucogingival problems are:
1. Pockets extending up to or beyond mucogingival junction.
2. Recession causing denudation of root surfaces.
3. High frenum and muscle attachments.
4. Inadequate width of attached gingiva.

Q4. What are the objectives of mucogingival surgery?

Answer

1. Widening the zone of attached gingiva.
2. Coverage of denuded roots.
3. Removal of aberrant frenum.
4. Creation of some vestibular depth when it is lacking.
5. As an adjunct to routine pocket elimination procedures.

Q5. What are the indications for mucogingival surgery?

Answer

1. Augmentation of the edentulous ridge.
2. Prevention of ridge collapse associated with tooth extraction.
3. Crown lengthening.
4. Loss of interdental papilla, which presents as esthetic and/or phonetic defect.

Q6. What are the techniques used to increase the width of attached gingiva?

Answer

The techniques used to increase the width of attached gingiva are:
1. Gingival extension operation by free soft tissue autograft.
2. Apical displacement of the pocket wall and other techniques like fenestration operation and vestibular extension operation.

Q7. What are the advantages of free soft tissue autograft?

Answer

1. High degree of predictability—only with increasing width of keratinized gingiva.
2. Simplicity.
3. Ability to treat multiple teeth at the same time.
4. This procedure can be performed where there is inadequate keratinized gingiva adjacent to the involved area.

Q8. What are the disadvantages of free soft tissue autograft?

Answer

1. Two operative sites.
2. Compromised blood supply.
3. Greater discomfort.
4. Lack of predictability in attempting root coverage.

Q9. What are the indications for free soft tissue autograft?

Answer

1. An inadequate zone of attached gingiva.
2. Abnormal muscle attachment.

3. Shallow vestibular depth.
4. Gingival recession.
5. Deep pockets to prevent rapid initial down growth of epithelium.

Q10. What is the ideal graft thickness?
Answer

Thin or intermediate thickness graft is best for increasing the zone of attached gingiva (0.5–0.75 mm).

Thick or full thickness graft is indicated for root coverage and ridge augmentation.

Q11. What are the donor sites for free gingival graft?
Answer

Donor tissue is obtained from, edentulous ridge area, but the ideal and most common site is the palatal mucosa.

Q12. What are the other techniques used for widening of attached gingiva?
Answer

1. Fenestration operation/periosteal separation.
2. Vestibular extension operation.

Q13. What are the advantages of root coverage procedures?
Answer

1. Reduces root sensitivity.
2. Improves esthetics.
3. Manage the defects resulting from root caries removal and/or cervical abrasions.
4. Manage mucogingival defect, which fail to respond to altering abusive toothbrushing techniques and/or plaque removal.

Q14. Classify gingival recession.
Answer

Sullivan and Atkins classified isolated gingival recession into four types:
1. Shallow-narrow.
2. Shallow-wide.
3. Deep-narrow.
4. Deep-wide.

Miller's Classification

Class I: Marginal tissue recession that does not extend to the mucogingival junction. There is no loss of bone or soft tissue in the interdental area. This type of recession can be narrow or wide.

Class II: Marginal tissue recession that extends to or beyond the mucogingival junction. There is no loss of bone and soft tissue in the interdental area. This type of recession may be wide or narrow.

Class III: Marginal tissue recession that extends to or beyond the mucogingival junction. In addition, there is bone and/or soft tissue loss interdentally or tooth may be malposed.

Class IV: Marginal tissue recession extends to or beyond the mucogingival junction with severe bone and soft tissue loss interdentally and/or severe tooth malposition.

Q15. What is the prognosis of gingival recession?
Answer

Type of recession prognosis:
1. Class I and II—good to excellent.
2. Class III—only partial coverage can be expected.
3. Class IV—very poor.

Q16. What are the procedures for root coverage?
Answer

Procedures for root coverage can be divided into:
1. Conventional procedures.
2. Regenerative procedures.

Q17. What are the conventional root coverage procedures?
Answer

Conventional Procedures

Depending on the width of the attached gingiva, i.e. if adequate width is present at the donor site, the following procedures can be selected:
1. Laterally (horizontally) displaced flap.
2. Double papilla flap.
3. Coronally positioned flap.

If the donor site is associated with inadequate width:
1. Free soft tissue autograft.
2. Subepithelial connective tissue grafts are available.

Regenerative Procedures

Guided tissue regeneration (GTR) has been proposed.

Q18. Who developed sliding flap operation?
Answer

In 1956, Grupe and Warren developed an original and unique procedure called sliding flap operation.

Q19. What are the advantages of laterally displaced flap?
Answer

1. One surgical site.
2. Good vascularity of the pedicle flap.
3. Ability to cover isolated, denuded roots that have adequate donor tissue laterally.

Q20. What are the disadvantages of laterally displaced flap?

Answer

1. Limited by the amount of adjacent keratinized attached gingiva.
2. Possibility of recession at the donor site.
3. Dehiscence or fenestration at the donor site.
4. Limited to one or two teeth with gingival recession.

Q21. What are the indications for a laterally displaced flap?

Answer

1. For covering the isolated denuded root.
2. When there is sufficient width of interdental papilla in the adjacent teeth.
3. Sufficient vestibular depth.

Q22. What are the contraindications for a laterally displaced flap?

Answer

1. Presence of deep interproximal pockets.
2. Excessive root prominence.
3. Deep or extensive root abrasion or erosion.
4. Significant loss of interproximal bone height.

Q23. Who described double papilla flap?

Answer

First described by Wainberg as the double lateral repositioned flap and was refined by Cohen and Ross as the double papilla flap.

Q24. What are the indications for a double papilla flap?

Answer

1. When the interproximal papillae adjacent to the mucogingival problem are sufficiently wide.
2. When the attached gingiva on an approximating tooth is insufficient to allow for a lateral pedicle flap.
3. When periodontal pockets are not present.

Q25. What are the advantages of a double papilla flap?

Answer

1. The risk of loss of alveolar bone is minimized because the interdental bone is more resistant to loss, than radicular bone.
2. The papillae usually supply a greater width of attached gingiva, than from the radicular surface of a tooth.
3. The clinical predictability of this procedure is fairly good.

Q26. What are the disadvantages of a double papilla flap?

Answer

Technique sensitive—having tendency to join together the small flap in such a way so that they act as a single flap.

Q27. What are the indications for a coronally repositioned flap?

Answer

1. Esthetic coverage of exposed roots.
2. For tooth sensitivity owing to gingival recession.

Q28. What are the advantages of a coronally repositioned flap?

Answer

1. Treatment of multiple areas of root exposure.
2. No need for involvement of adjacent teeth.
3. High degree of success.
4. Even if the procedure does not work, it does not increase the existing problem.

Q29. What are the disadvantages of a coronally repositioned flap?

Answer

There is a need for two surgical procedures, if the zone of keratinized gingiva is inadequate.

Q30. What are the indications for semilunar flap?

Answer: Areas where gingival recession is only 2–3 mm.

Q31. What are the advantages of a semilunar flap?

Answer

1. No vestibular shortening, as occurs with the coronally positioned flap.
2. No esthetic compromise of interproximal papillae.
3. No need for sutures.

Q32. What are the disadvantages of a semilunar flap?

Answer

1. Inability to treat large areas of gingival recession.
2. The need for a free gingival graft, if there is an underlying dehiscence or fenestration.

Q33. Who proposed the free gingival autograft?

Answer

In 1985, Miller applied this with few modifications to cover the denuded roots.

Q34. Who proposed the subepithelial connective tissue graft?

Answer

Proposed by Langer and Langer in 1985. In 1994, Bruno described modification of the original Langer and Langer technique.

Q35. What are the indications for a subepithelial connective tissue graft?

Answer

1. Where esthetics is of prime concern.
2. For covering multiple denuded roots.
3. In the absence of sufficient width of attached gingiva in the adjacent areas.

Q36. What are the advantages of a subepithelial connective tissue graft?

Answer

1. High degree of cosmetic enhancement.
2. Incurs no additional cost for autogenous donor tissue.
3. One step procedure.
4. Minimal palatal trauma.
5. Increased graft vascularity.

Q37. What are the disadvantages of a subepithelial connective tissue graft?

Answer

1. High degree of technical skills required.
2. Complicated suturing.

Q38. What are the modifications in the recipient site preparation in the subepithelial connective tissue graft procedure?

Answer

Envelope Technique

In this technique, first eliminate the sulcular epithelium by an internal bevel incision. Secondly, an 'envelope' is prepared apically and laterally to the recession by split incision.

Langer's Technique

In addition to the horizontal incision, two vertical releasing incisions 1–2 mm away from the gingival margin, extending one-half to one tooth wider mesiodistally, than the area of gingival recession is given.

Pouch and Tunnel Technique

In case of multiple adjacent recessions, 'envelopes' are prepared on each tooth for receiving connective tissue graft.

Q39. How is the graft procured from the donor site?

Answer

In the palate, a partial thickness flap is raised with two vertical releasing incisions; followed by this, the connective tissue is harvested by placing two horizontal and two vertical incisions to the bone. After the graft removal, the flap is positioned back and sutured.

Q40. What are the indications for root coverage GTR technique?

Answer

1. Esthetic demand.
2. Indicated for single tooth with wide, deep localized recessions.
3. For areas of root sensitivity where oral hygiene is impaired.
4. For repair of recessions associated with failing or unesthetic class V restorations.

Q41. What are the advantages of guided tissue regeneration for root coverage procedure?

Answer

1. Techniques do not require a secondary donor surgical site, reducing postoperative discomfort.
2. New tissue blends evenly with the adjacent tissue, providing highly esthetic results.

Q42. What are the disadvantages of GTR for root coverage?

Answer

1. It is a sensitive technique.
2. Insurance of additional cost of barrier membrane.

Q43. What are the modifications in GTR technique for root coverage procedure?

Answer

1. Titanium-reinforced membranes are used to create the space below the membrane.
2. Resorbable membranes have been used to prevent a second surgery.

Q44. What is a frenum?
Answer

A frenum is a fold of mucous membrane usually with enclosed muscle fibers that attaches the lips and cheeks to the alveolar mucosa and/or gingiva and underlying periosteum.

Q45. What is frenectomy?
Answer

It is the complete removal of frenum including its attachment to the bone. It is indicated for the correction of abnormal diastema.

Q46. What is frenotomy?
Answer

It is the incision and relocation of the frenum to create a zone of attached gingiva between the gingival margin and the frenum (suffices for periodontal problems).

Q47. What are the types of frenal attachments?
Answer

Frenal attachment may be of four types:
1. *Papillary:* Where the frenum is inserted into the interdental papilla.
2. *Mucosal type:* Where the frenum is attached in the alveolar mucosa.
3. *Papillary penetrating types:* Where the frenum is inserted from the facial to palatal papilla.
4. *Gingival:* Where the frenum is in the attached gingiva.

Q48. What does periodontal plastic surgery include?
Answer

In 1996, World Workshop in clinical periodontics renamed mucogingival surgery as 'periodontal plastic surgery' and broadened to include the following problems:
1. Lack of sufficient vestibular depth.
2. Inadequate crown length for restorative procedures.
3. Denuded root surface.
4. Alveolar defects.
5. Open gingival embrasures.
6. Excessive gingival pigmentation.
7. Aberrant frenum.
8. Inadequate attached gingiva.
9. Impacted/unerupted teeth requiring orthodontic treatment.
10. Excessive gingival display and gingival asymmetry.

Q49. Who proposed vestibular extension technique?
Answer

The 'vestibular extension technique', was originally described by Edlan and Mejchar. Currently, this technique is of historical interest only.

CHAPTER 47

Furcation Involvement and its Management

Q1. What is furcation involvement?

Answer

Furcation involvement refers to commonly occurring conditions in which the bifurcations and trifurcations of multirooted teeth are invaded by the disease process.

Q2. Define furcation.

Answer

According to American Academy of Periodontology (2001), it is defined as pathologic resorption of bone within the furcation.

Q3. What is the primary etiologic factor for furcation?

Answer

Bacterial plaque and long-standing inflammation of periodontal tissues.

Q4. What are the anatomic considerations in furcation defects?

Answer

1. Root trunk length.
2. Root separation.
3. The surface of the tooth just coronal to the root separation. This area is usually concave, grooved or fluted.
4. The roof of furcation, which contains furcation ridges. These ridges run mesiodistally in lower and buccolingually in upper molars.

Q5. What are the anatomic considerations of tooth in furcation defects?

Answer

1. Root trunk length.
2. Concavity of the inner surface of exposed roots.
3. Degree of separation of roots/inter-radicular dimension.
4. Cervical enamel projections.
5. Anatomy of the furcation.
6. Presence of accessory pulpal canals.

Q6. Classify cervical enamel projections.

Answer

It was classified by Masters and Hoskins in 1964 as:
1. *Grade I:* The enamel projection extends from the cementoenamel junction of the tooth toward the furcation entrance.
2. *Grade II:* The enamel projection approaches the entrance to the furcation, but does not enter the furcation and hence has no horizontal component.
3. *Grade III:* The enamel projection extends horizontally into the furcation.

Q7. What are the anatomic considerations of bone?

Answer

Bone shape in the exposed furcation area has a horizontal component that determines the grades (I, II and III) of the involvement and a vertical component that most often creates a depression in the center of the remaining bone, similar to a crater in an interdental area. The vertical component can also appear as a vertical or angular loss toward one of the roots. The latter defect can have one, two or three osseous walls or can be funnel-shaped around one root.

Q8. What are the considerations of gingival management in furcation area?

Answer

The presence of sufficient attached keratinized gingival tissue and adequate vestibular depth will facilitate the gingival management of the furcation area.

Q9. Classify furcation involvement given by Glickman.

Answer

Glickman in 1953 had classified furcation involvement into the following:

1. *Grade I:* It is the incipient or early lesion. The pocket is suprabony, involving soft tissue. There is slight bone loss in the furcation area. No radiographic changes.
2. *Grade II:* In this type, bone is destroyed on one or more aspects of the furcation, but a portion of alveolar bone and periodontal ligament remains intact, permitting only partial penetration of the probe into the furcation. The lesion is essentially a cul-de-sac. The radiograph may or may not reveal the grade II involvement.
3. *Grade III:* In this type, the inter-radicular bone is completely lost, but the facial or lingual surfaces are occluded by gingival tissues. Therefore, the furcation opening cannot be seen clinically, but it is essentially a through-and-through tunnel. If the radiographs are taken with proper angulation and the roots are divergent, the lesion will appear as a radiolucent area between the roots.
4. *Grade IV:* As in grade III lesions, the inter-radicular bone is completely lost, but in grade IV involvement, the gingival tissues recede apically, so that the furcation opening is seen clinically. The radiographic changes are essentially the same as that of grade III lesion.

Q10. Classify furcation based on the vertical component.

Answer

Based on Vertical Component (Tarnow and Fletcher in 1984)

Depending on the distance from the base of the defect to the roof of the furcation, they can be classified as:
1. *Subgroup A:* Vertical destruction of bone up to one-third of the inter-radicular height (0–3 mm).
2. *Subgroup B:* Vertical destruction of bone up to two-third of the inter-radicular height (4–7 mm).
3. *Subgroup C:* Vertical destruction beyond the apical-third (7 mm or more).

Q11. Classify furcation based on the horizontal component.

Answer

Furcations can be classified as:
1. *Degree I:* Horizontal bone loss of less than 3 mm.
2. *Degree II:* Horizontal bone loss of more than 3 mm.
3. *Degree III:* Through-and-through horizontal lesion.

Q12. How is a furcation detected?

Answer

Furcation can be clinically detected by using Nabers probe along with a simultaneous blast of warm air to facilitate visualization and radiographs also help detect the furcation invasions.

Q13. Classify furcation according to Goldman.

Answer

According to Goldman (1958):
1. *Grade I:* Incipient.
2. *Grade II:* Cul-de-sac.
3. *Grade III:* Through-and-through.

Q14. Classify furcation as given by Ramfjord and Ash.

Answer

According to Ramfjord and Ash (1979):
1. *Class I:* Beginning involvement. Tissue destruction less than 2 mm (i.e. less than one-third tooth width).
2. *Class II:* Cul-de-sac. Tissue destruction more than 2 mm (i.e. more than one-third tooth width), but not through-and-through.
3. *Class III:* Through-and-through involvement.

Q15. Classify furcation according to Fedi.

Answer

According to Fedi (1985), it is a combination of Glickman's and Hamp's classification:
1. *Grade I:* It is the incipient or early lesion. The pocket is suprabony, involving soft tissue. There is slight bone loss in the furcation area. No radiographic changes.
2. *Grade II:* In grade II cases, bone is destroyed on one or more aspects of the furcation, but a portion of alveolar bone and periodontal ligament remains intact, permitting only partial penetration of the probe into the furcation. The lesion is essentially a cul-de-sac. The radiograph may or may not reveal the grade II involvement. It can be further divided into:
   a. *Degree I:* Inter-radicular bone loss less than 3 mm.
   b. *Degree II:* Inter-radicular bone loss more than 3 mm.
   c. Grade III and grade IV are same as Glickman's classifications.

Q16. What are the clinical features of furcation defects?

Answer

1. The mandibular first molars are the most common sites and maxillary premolars are the least common.
2. The denuded furcation may be visible clinically or covered by the wall of the pocket.
3. Associated with suprabony and infrabony pockets.
4. Periodontal abscess.
5. Root caries and tooth mobility are common.

Q17. What are the microscopic features of furcation defects?

Answer

1. Rootward extension of the periodontal pocket.
2. In its early stages, there is a widening of the periodontal space with cellular and inflammatory fluid exudation,

followed by epithelial proliferation into the furcation area from an adjoining periodontal pocket.
3. Extension of the inflammation into the bone leads to resorption and reduction in bone height.
4. The bone destructive pattern may produce horizontal loss or there may be angular osseous defects associated with infrabony pockets. Plaque, calculus and bacterial debris occupy the denuded furcation space.

Q18. What is the prognosis of furcation defects in maxillary teeth?

Answer

1. *Maxillary first premolar:* Poor prognosis.
2. *Maxillary molars:* Not Good.
3. *Mandibular molars:* Good.

Q19. Why is the prognosis poor for maxillary first premolars?

Answer

Maxillary first premolar often shows fusion of the roots and the furcation area may be located very much apically and also the roots of the maxillary first premolars are placed buccally and palatally with furcation opening in a mesiodistal direction. For these reasons, furcation involvement in maxillary first premolar has poor prognosis.

Q20. Why is the prognosis not good in maxillary molars?

Answer

In maxillary molars, furcations may open buccally, mesially and distally because of the presence of the three roots. Since access from proximal areas is difficult for plaque control, prognosis of furcation involvement in maxillary molars is not good.

Q21. Why do mandibular molars have good prognosis in furcation involvement?

Answer

Mandibular molars have two roots, placed mesially and distally, and the furcation opens buccolingually. The roots are usually divergent especially in mandibular first molars. As a result, prognosis of furcation involvement in mandibular molar (especially the first molar) is considered good.

Q22. What are the treatment modalities for furcation defects?

Answer

Two treatment modalities have been proposed:
1. Traditional treatment procedures.
2. Reconstructive or regenerative treatment.

Q23. What factors should be considered for deciding the mode of therapy?

Answer

Factors to be considered when deciding on a mode of therapy are as follows:
1. Degree of involvement.
2. Crown-root ratio.
3. Length of roots.
4. Degree of root separation.
5. Strategic value of the tooth or teeth in question.
6. Root anatomy of the involved tooth.
7. Residual tooth mobility.
8. Endodontic therapy and complications.
9. Ability to eliminate the defect.
10. Periodontal condition of the adjacent teeth.

Q24. What is the traditional treatment procedure?

Answer

They are those which are directed to maintain the state of the health, but do not attempt to regenerate the lost periodontium. The goal is to prevent the further progression of the disease and provide an environment, which will help in adequate plaque control.

Q25. What is the traditional treatment procedure for a grade I furcation defect?

Answer

Grade I: They are usually associated with suprabony pockets, hence:
1. Initial preparation or scaling and root planing.
2. Curettage or gingivectomy to expose the furcation area.
3. Odontoplasty to reshape the facial groove in order to prevent plaque accumulation.

Q26. What is the traditional treatment procedure for a grade II furcation defect?

Answer

In shallow grade II invasions:
1. Osteoplasty with limited ostectomy may be helpful.
2. Odontoplasty can be performed.

In severe grades II to IV invasions, elimination of furcation by:
1. Root resection or amputation.
2. Hemisection or root separation.
3. Bicuspidization/root separation.
4. Tunnel preparation.

Q27. How are the grade III and grade IV furcation defects treated?

Answer

Grade III and grade IV can be treated with root resection and root separation.

Q28. Enumerate the regenerative treatment procedures for furcation defects.

Answer

Grade I: Traditional treatment will do.

Grade II: Various regenerative techniques include:
1. Autogenous bone grafting, e.g. osseous coagulum, bone blend.
2. Allografts, e.g. freeze-dried bone allografts (FDBA), demineralized freeze-dried bone allografts, DFDBA).
3. Alloplasts—hydroxyapatite, tricalcium phosphate.
4. Citric acid root conditioning with coronally positioned flap.
5. Guided tissue regeneration and combination techniques.

For grade III and grade IV furcation involvements, the success rate is limited.

Q29. What is root resection or amputation?

Answer

It is the surgical removal of all or a portion of the root before or after endodontic treatment.

Q30. What is hemisection or root separation?

Answer

It is the surgical removal of a root with the associated part of the crown. It is frequently used with reference to lower molars.

Q31. What is bicuspidization?

Answer

Root separation/bicuspidization is the sectioning of the root complex and the maintenance of all roots.

Q32. What is tunnel preparation?

Answer

It is by transforming the grade II lesion to grades III and IV for better access, but it is not performed anymore because of increased incidence of root caries.

Q33. What are the indications for root resection and root separation?

Answer

1. Severe bone loss affecting one or more roots untreatable with regenerative procedures.
2. Class II or III furcation invasions or involvement.
3. Severe recession or dehiscence of a root.

Q34. What are the contraindications for root resection and root separation?

Answer

1. General contraindications like systemic diseases and poor oral hygiene.
2. Fused roots, unfavorable tissue architecture.
3. Roots that are endodontically untreatable.

Q35. What are the phases of treatment for root resection and root separation?

Answer

1. Endodontic phase.
2. Restorative phase.
3. Surgical phase.

Q36. What are the advantages of the endodontic phase of treatment?

Answer

1. Better bone recontouring during surgery.
2. Allows precise flap closure.
3. Easy adaptation for temporary prosthesis.

Q37. Which is the most commonly resected root?

Answer

Most commonly, distobuccal root of the maxillary first molar is resected.

Q38. What is root complex?

Answer

It is the portion of a tooth that is located apical to the cementoenamel junction (CEJ).

Q39. What are the parts of root complex?

Answer

The root complex may be divided into two parts:
1. The root trunk.
2. The root cones.

Q40. What is root trunk?

Answer

Root trunk represents the undivided region of the root, which is the distance between the CEJ and the separation line between the roots.

Q41. What is root cone?

Answer

Root cone is present within the divided region of the root complex. Two or more root cones make up the furcation region.

Q42. What is furcation fornix?

Answer

Furcation fornix is the roof of the furcation.

Q43. What is divergence?

Answer

Divergence is the distance between two roots, which normally increases in apical direction.

Q44. What is coefficient of separation?

Answer

Coefficient of separation is the length of the root cones in relation to the length of the root complex.

Q45. What are the methods used to diagnose furcation?

Answer

1. Probing.
2. Radiographs.

Q46. How a furcation is detected using a probe?

Answer

1. Furcation is detected using a curved graduated periodontal probe (Nabers probe), an explorer or a small curette, furcations can be identified.
2. Maxillary molars—mesial furcation entrance is located closer to palatal than to the buccal surface, hence, the mesial furcation should be probed from the palatal aspect of the tooth. Whereas the distal furcation is in the midway between buccal and palatal surfaces, hence, this furcation can be probed either from the buccal or palatal surface. The distal maxillary furcation is most frequently involved.

CHAPTER 48

Pulpoperiodontal Problems

Q1. What is retrograde periodontitis?
Answer

Periodontitis caused by pulpal infections that have entered the periodontal ligament either through the apical foramen or through the lateral canals. Such a periodontal lesion is termed as 'retrograde periodontitis'.

Q2. Classify the pathways of communication between pulp and periodontium.
Answer

It can be classified into three categories:
1. Pathways of developmental origin:
   a. Apical foramen.
   b. Accessory canals and lateral canals.
   c. Developmental grooves.
   d. Enamel projections and pearls at the cervical portion.
2. Pathways of pathologic origin:
   a. Tooth fracture (vertical).
   b. Idiopathic resorption can be:
      - *Internal:* From the pulp to the surface of the tooth
      - *External:* From the external surface of the root to the pulp.
        Both internal and external resorption produces communication.
   c. Loss of cementum due to external irritants.
3. Pathways of iatrogenic origin:
   a. Exposure of dentinal tubules following root planing.
   b. Accidental lateral perforation during endodontic procedure.
   c. Root fracture due to endodontic procedure.

Q3. What are the causes of pulpal inflammation?
Answer

1. Instrumentation during periodontal, restorative or prosthetic procedures.
2. Progression of dental caries.
3. Tooth fractures.

Q4. Classify endoperiolesions.
Answer

Based on the etiology, diagnosis, prognosis and treatment, endoperiolesions can be classified into five groups:
1. Primary endodontic lesion.
2. Primary endodontic with secondary periodontal lesion.
3. Primary periodontal lesion.
4. Primary periodontal lesion with secondary endodontic involvement.
5. True combined lesions.

Q5. What are the bacteria found in endoperiolesions?
Answer

Bacteroides forsythus, *Porphyromonas gingivalis* and *Treponema denticola*, fusobacteria, spirochetes, *Wolinella* and *Peptostreptococcus* have been found in endoperiolesions.

Q6. What are the methods used in the diagnosis of endoperiolesions?
Answer

Radiographic analysis with gutta-percha tracing, periodontal probing and fiberoptic illumination to rule out a fracture that exists with vitality test and percussion tests.

Q7. What are the newer diagnostic methods for endoperiolesions?

Answer

Doppler devices, pulse oximetry and magnetic resonance imaging.

Q8. What is the drawback of vitality test in endoperiolesion?

Answer

Numerous studies have demonstrated the inaccuracy of vitality testing probably because pulp testing only indicates the neural response and gives little information about the vascularity or true vitality of the pulp.

Q9. Classify endoperiolesion according to Oliet and Pollock.

Answer

According to Oliet and Pollock (1968), based on treatment procedure:
1. Lesion that require endodontic treatment procedures only.
2. Lesion that require periodontal treatment procedures only.
3. Lesions that require combined endodontic-periodontic treatment procedures.

Q10. Classify endoperiolesions according to Weine.

Answer

According to Weine (1972):
1. *Class I:* Tooth in which symptoms clinically and radiographically simulate periodontal disease, but are infact due to pulpal inflammation and/or necrosis.
2. *Class II:* Tooth that has both pulpal or periapical disease and periodontal disease concomitantly.
3. *Class III:* Tooth that has no pulpal problem, but requires endodontic therapy plus root amputation to gain periodontal healing.
4. *Class IV:* Tooth that clinically and radiographically simulates pulpal or periapical disease, but infact has periodontal disease.

CHAPTER 49

Splints in Periodontal Therapy

Q1. Define dental splinting.
Answer

It is defined as the joining of two or more teeth into a rigid unit by means of a fixed or removable restorations/devices. Splint, by definition, is an appliance used for immobilization of injured or diseased parts.

Q2. What is periodontal splint?
Answer

It is an appliance used for maintaining or stabilizing mobile teeth in their functional position. The main objective of splinting is to promote healing and to increase the patient's comfort and function.

Q3. What are the objectives of splinting?
Answer

1. Provides rest.
2. *For redirection of forces:* The forces of occlusion are redirected in a more axial direction over all the teeth included in the splint.
3. *For redistribution of forces:* Redistribution ensures that forces do not exceed the adaptive capacity of the periodontium.
4. *To preserve arch integrity:* Splinting restores proximal contacts, reducing food impaction and consequent breakdown of the periodontium.
5. *Restoration of functional stability:* Restores a functional occlusion, stabilizes mobile abutment teeth and increases masticatory efficiency.
6. *Psychological well-being:* Gives the patient freedom from mobile teeth, thereby giving a sense of well-being.
7. *To stabilize mobile teeth during surgical therapy:* Especially regenerative one.
8. To prevent the eruption of teeth without an antagonist.

Q4. Classify splints.
Answer

1. According to the period of stabilization:
   a. Temporary stabilization.
   b. Provisional stabilization.
   c. Permanent splints.
2. According to the type of material:
   a. Bonded, composite resin button splint.
   b. Braided wire splint.
   c. A-splints.
3. According to the location on the tooth:
   a. Intracoronal:
      - Composite resin with wire
      - Inlays
      - Nylon wire.
   b. Extracoronal:
      - Tooth-bonded plastic
      - Night guard
      - Welded bands.

Q5. What are the various splints commonly used?
Answer

1. Splints for anterior teeth:
   a. Direct bonding system using acid-etch techniques and a light cured resin.
   b. Intracoronal wire and acrylic wire resin splint—it involves the teeth with stainless steel wire placed in the slots thus stabilizing the teeth.
2. Splints for posterior teeth:
   a. Intracoronal amalgam wire splints—it uses resin restoration with wire on the proximal amalgam restored areas of the tooth.
   b. Bite guard.
   c. Rigid occlusal splint.
   d. Composite splint.

Q6. What are the principles of splinting?

Answer

1. *Inclusion of sufficient number of healthy teeth:* It is suggested that the healthy teeth included in the splint should have double the root surface area of the mobile teeth to be splinted. Since the posterior teeth are multirooted, the number of healthy teeth to be included in the splint in the posterior segment will be less as compared to the anterior.
2. *Splint around the arch:* Muscles of the lips, cheek and tongue exert some forces on the teeth. Based on the direction of such forces applied on the teeth, the dental arch can be divided into two posterior sextants and an anterior sextant. In the posterior sextant, the tongue pushes the teeth buccally and the muscles of the cheek counteract it by pushing them lingually. When the splint is confined to any one sextant, the splinted teeth tend to tilt lingually or outwards depending on the muscular forces. Such a collapse of the splinted sextant can be prevented by including few teeth from the adjacent sextant. This is termed splinting around the arch.
3. Coronoplasty may be performed to relieve traumatic occlusion.
4. The splint should be fabricated in such a way as to facilitate proper plaque control.
5. Splint should be esthetically acceptable and should not interfere with occlusion.

Q7. What are the indications for splinting?

Answer

1. It stabilizes moderate to advanced tooth mobility that cannot be reduced by other means and which has not responded to occlusal adjustment and periodontal therapy.
2. When it interferes with normal masticatory function.
3. Facilitates scaling and surgical procedures.
4. Stabilizes teeth after orthodontic movement.
5. Stabilizes teeth after acute dental trauma, e.g. subluxation, avulsion, etc.
6. In order to prevent tipping and drifting of teeth.
7. Prevent extrusion of unopposed teeth.

Q8. What are the contraindications for splinting?

Answer

1. Moderate to severe tooth mobility in the presence of periodontal inflammation and/or primary occlusal trauma.
2. Insufficient number of firm/sufficiently firm teeth to stabilize mobile teeth.
3. Prior occlusal adjustment has not been done on teeth with occlusal trauma or occlusal interference.
4. Patient not maintaining oral hygiene.

CHAPTER 50

Dental Implants: Periodontal Considerations

Q1. Define oral implantology.

Answer

Oral implantology is the science and discipline concerned with the diagnosis, design, insertion, restoration and for management of alloplastic or autogenous oral structures to restore the loss of contour, comfort, function, esthetics, speech and/or health of the partially or completely edentulous patient.

Q2. Define osseointegration.

Answer

Direct structural and functional connection between ordered living bone and the surface of the load carrying implant.

Q3. What are the different bone implant interfaces?

Answer

The relationship between endosseous implants and bone involves mechanisms like:
1. Fibro-osseous integration.
2. Osseointegration.
3. Bioactive integration.

Q4. What are the different biomaterials used for implants?

Answer

1. Metals and alloys.
2. Inert ceramics.
3. Calcium phosphate ceramics.
4. Polymers.

Q5. What are the basic types of implants?

Answer

Based on the Shape and Form

1. Endosteal.
2. Subperiosteal.
3. Transosteal.
4. Intramucosal inserts/submucosal implants/subdermal implants.
5. Endodontic stabilizer.

Q6. What are the absolute contraindications for implant therapy?

Answer

1. Uncontrolled diabetes mellitus.
2. Long-term immunosuppressant drug therapy.
3. Diseases of connective tissue.
4. Blood dyscrasias and coagulopathies.
5. Regional malignancy.
6. Metastatic disease.
7. Previous radiation to the jaws that might lead to postsurgical osteoradionecrosis.
8. Alcohol or drug addiction.
9. Severe psychologic disorders.

Q7. What are the absolute requirements for providing implant therapy to a patient?

Answer

1. Have an acceptable patient.
2. Implant made of biocompatible material.
3. Be durable.
4. Have proper surface quality.
5. Have acceptable socket created in bone.
6. Have surgical procedure properly done.
7. Have healing completed with acceptable bone interface.
8. Have healing period without pathological stress.
9. Have normal implant function without pathological stress.

Q8. What are the different types of peri-implant diseases?

Answer

1. *Peri-implant mucositis:* Inflammatory changes, which are confined to soft tissue surrounding an implant is termed as peri-implant mucositis.

2. *Peri-implantitis:* It is a progressive peri-implant bone loss in conjunction with soft tissue inflammatory lesion. Peri-implantitis begins at the coronal portion of the implant, while the more apical portion of implant remains osseointegrated. This means that the implant is not clinically mobile until late stages when bone loss has progressed to involve the complete implant surface.

Maintenance Phase (Supportive Periodontal Treatment)

Q1. What is the importance of maintenance therapy?

Answer

Maintenance therapy is often supportive in nature; hence, it is also known as supportive periodontal treatment (SPT). In this phase, patients must be made to understand the purpose of a maintenance program and the dentist must emphasize on the fact that the preservation of the teeth in question are dependent on it.

Q2. What is the rationale for supportive periodontal therapy?

Answer

Rationale for maintenance phase is to prevent or minimize the recurrence of periodontal diseases by controlling factors known to contribute to the disease process. The main aim of long-term therapy is to provide supervised control for the patient in order to maintain a healthy and functional natural dentition for life. It is only with proper maintenance, including early detection and treatment of recurrent periodontal diseases that such an objective can be achieved.

Q3. What are the causes for recurrence of periodontal disease?

Answer

1. Incomplete subgingival plaque removal.
2. Nature of dentogingival unit.
3. Improper restorations placed after the periodontal treatment was completed.
4. Failure of the patient to return for periodic recall visits.
5. Presence of some systemic diseases that may affect host resistance to previously acceptable levels of plaque.

Q4. What are the goals of supportive periodontal treatment?

Answer

1. To prevent or minimize the recurrence and progression of periodontal disease in patients who have been previously treated for gingivitis, periodontitis and for peri-implantitis.
2. To prevent or reduce the incidence of tooth loss by monitoring the dentition and by any prosthetic replacement of the natural teeth.
3. To increase the probability and treating in a timely manner, other diseases or conditions found in the oral cavity.

Q5. What are the objectives of maintenance phase?

Answer

1. Preservation of alveolar bone support (radiographically).
2. Maintenance of stable, clinical attachment level.
3. Reinforcement and re-evaluation of proper home care.
4. Maintenance of a healthy and functional oral environment.

Q6. What is the sequence of maintenance visits?

Answer

Schallhorn and Snider (1981) proposed four separate categories of periodontal maintenance therapy. They are:

1. *Preventive maintenance therapy:* Periodontally healthy individuals.
2. *Trial maintenance therapy:* Mild to moderate periodontitis.
3. *Compromised maintenance therapy:* Medically compromised patients where active therapy is not possible.

4. *Postmaintenance treatment therapy:* Maintenance for prevention of recurrence of disease.

Q7. What are the procedures to be performed at the time of recall?

Answer

Procedure evaluation
1. *At clinical examination:* All findings recorded at the baseline are compared evaluations of complete oral and periodontal status, occlusal and prosthetic appliances, etc.
2. *Radiographically:* Assessment of bone levels and any additional findings are recorded.
3. *Assessment of disease:* By comparing the findings obtained at base line.
4. *Assessment of patient's oral hygiene:* Comparison with baseline data and behavioral modification if necessary.
5. *Treatment:* Removal of any fresh deposits, occlusal therapy, application of antimicrobial agents if indicated. Appointments for future periodontal therapy.

CHAPTER 52

Occlusal Evaluation and Therapy in the Management of Periodontal Disease

Q1. What is occlusion?

Answer

It is defined as the functional relationship between the components of the masticatory system including the teeth, supporting tissues, neuromuscular system, temporomandibular joints and craniofacial skeleton.

Q2. What is intercuspal position (ICP)?

Answer

The position of the mandible when there is maximal intercuspation between the maxillary and mandibular teeth.

Q3. What is excursive movement?

Answer

Any movement of the mandible away from ICP.

Q4. What is protrusion?

Answer

Movement of the mandible anteriorly from ICP.

Q5. What is retrusion?

Answer

Movement of the mandible posteriorly from ICP.

Q6. What is a physiologic occlusion?

Answer

It is when no signs of dysfunction or disease are present and no treatment is indicated.

Q7. What is a non-physiologic (or traumatic) occlusion?

Answer

It is associated with dysfunction or disease due to tissue injury and treatment may be indicated.

Q8. What is a therapeutic occlusion?

Answer

It is the result of specific interventions designed to treat dysfunction or disease.

Q9. Describe the management of trauma from occlusion.

Answer

1. In cases of primary occlusal trauma with gingivitis or periodontitis, the treatment is simple and conservative. First, periodontal therapy is done, which include plaque control, scaling and root planing. If there is progressive mobility, then occlusal therapy in the form of selective grinding and the use of night guard may be justified.
2. In cases of secondary occlusal trauma and advanced periodontitis, the treatment is often complicated. It often requires advanced periodontal therapy, including root resection, antimicrobial therapy and regenerative procedures along with adjunctive orthodontics, occlusal adjustment by selective grinding and splinting for periodontal stabilization is advocated.

Q10. What is occlusal therapy?

Answer

Occlusal therapy is performed to establish a stable functional relationship, favorable to the oral health of the patient, including the periodontium. Various procedures to achieve this objective are:
1. Interocclusal appliance therapy.
2. Occlusal adjustment.
3. Restorative procedures.
4. Orthodontic movement and orthognathic surgery.

Q11. What is coronoplasty?

Answer

Occlusal adjustment or coronoplasty is the selective reshaping of occlusal surface with the goal of establishing a stable, non-traumatic occlusion. This is achieved by reshaping the crown surfaces and eliminating undesirable occlusal supracontacts and the creation of a stable mandibular position. Coronoplasty is generally performed after gingival inflammation and periodontal pockets have been eliminated.

CHAPTER 53

The Role of Orthodontics as an Adjunct to Periodontal Therapy

Q1. What is the role of orthodontics as an adjunct to periodontal treatment?

Answer

The primary objective of periodontal therapy is to restore and maintain the health and integrity of the attachment apparatus of teeth. In adults, the loss of teeth or periodontal support can result in pathologic tooth migration involving either a single tooth or a group of teeth. This may result in the development of a median diastema or general spacing of the teeth, rotation or tipping of premolars and molars with the collapse of the posterior occlusion and decreasing vertical dimension. Adjunctive orthodontic therapy is necessary to resolve these problems.

Q2. What is the rationale for orthodontic treatment in periodontal therapy?

Answer

1. Reducing plaque retention.
2. Improving gingival and osseous forms.
3. Facilitating prosthetic replacements.
4. Improving esthetics.

Q3. How orthodontics can be used as an adjunct to overall treatment?

Answer

1. Uprighting or repositioning of teeth to improve parallelism of abutment teeth (e.g. tipped abutment teeth).
2. Improving future pontic spaces (e.g. inadequate spaces).
3. Correcting crossbites.
4. Extruding teeth/Intruding teeth.
5. Correcting crowding of teeth.
6. Achieving adequate embrasure space and proper root positioning.
7. Repositioning teeth for implant placement.
8. Restoring lost vertical dimension.
9. Increasing/decreasing overjet/overbite.
10. Closure of diastema.

Q4. What are the indications and contraindications of orthodontic therapy?

Answer

Indications

This includes common problems that can be solved by minor orthodontic therapy such as crowded teeth, closure of anterior diastema, mesial tilting of molars and open contacts.

Contraindications

The only contraindication is the persistence of active disease in spite of phase-I therapy procedures. The superimposition of tooth movement on inflamed gingiva may exacerbate the periodontal problem. This can occur by shifting the position of plaque subgingivally, increasing the rate of periodontal attachment loss and altering the morphology of the bone.

Q5. What should be the timing of orthodontic procedures in periodontal treatment?

Answer

It is generally recommended that orthodontics should be preceded by periodontal therapy based on the belief that orthodontics, in the presence of inflammation, can lead to rapid and irreversible breakdown of the periodontium. But any elimination procedures like pocket or osseous reduction procedures may be postponed until the end of orthodontic therapy because tooth movement may modify gingival and osseous morphology.

Q6. What are the iatrogenic effects associated with orthodontic treatment?

Answer

Orthodontic treatment may cause injuries to the teeth and periodontium, but in most of the cases, the changes are reversible and regeneration and repair of the tooth structures and periodontal tissues can occur. In some cases, the changes may get out of control resulting in irreparable damage. All the precautions should be taken to avoid this and radiography should be performed at regular intervals in order to disclose any iatrogenic effects during the orthodontic treatment.

Root Resorption

Some amount of root resorption is unavoidable, especially if it is seen at the marginal and middle thirds of the root, which can be repaired by apposition of cellular cementum.

Q7. What are the effects of orthodontic bands on the periodontium?

Answer

Short-term effects: Gingivitis and gingival hyperplasia, mostly not associated with loss of attachment.

Long-term effects: Loss of attachment, root resorption or no effects. Any of these three possibilities may be seen in adult patients.

Q8. What are the effects of orthodontics on dentition with normal height of attachment apparatus?

Answer

Orthodontic forces, cause no damage to the supra-alveolar connective tissue, and orthodontic treatment will therefore not result in periodontal tissue breakdown and pocket formation.

Q9. What are the effects of orthodontics on dentition with reduced height of attachment apparatus?

Answer

1. In the absence of plaque, orthodontic forces and tooth movements, failed to induce gingivitis, whereas in the presence of plaque, similar forces cause angular bone defects associated with attachment loss.
2. Orthodontic forces if kept within biologic limit, failed to cause gingival inflammation even in the regions with reduced periodontal support, but are of the non-inflammatory type.

Q10. Describe the microbiology around orthodontic bands.

Answer

1. Increased *Lactobacillus* count.
2. Increased motile organisms.
3. Increased anaerobes like *Prevotella intermedia*.
4. Decreased count of facultative microorganisms/anaerobes.

Q11. Describe the changes occurring after the force applied on bone.

Answer

When bone surrounding the tooth is subjected to a force, it responds in the following manner:

1. Resorption occurs where there is pressure and new bone forms where there is tension.
2. When pressure is applied to the tooth, there is an initial period of movement for 6–8 days, as the periodontal ligament is compressed. Compression of periodontal ligament results in blood supply being cut off to an area of the periodontal ligament and this produces an avascular, cell-free zone by a process termed 'hyalinization'. When hyalinization occurs, the tooth stops moving (depending on the forces). The hyalinized zone is eliminated by periodontal regeneration that occurs from the reorganization of the area through resorption by the marrow spaces (undermining resorption) and adjacent areas of unaffected periodontal ligament and alveolar bone. Once the hyalinized zone is removed, tooth movement can occur again. Regeneration of periodontal ligament does not occur when inflammation is present in periodontal tissue. Hence, the inflammation needs to be controlled by periodontal treatment.

CHAPTER 54

Periodontal-restorative Inter-relationship

Q1. Why is periodontal-restorative inter-relationship important?

Answer

For restorations to survive, long-term restorative procedures must be performed on a periodontium free of inflammation, pockets without any mucogingival involvement and with the contour and shape of the periodontium corrected for a good functional and esthetic restorative result. For the periodontium to remain healthy, restorations must be critically prepared so that, they will remain in harmony with the surrounding periodontal tissues.

Q2. What are the different margins of the restoration?

Answer

1. Supragingival.
2. Equigingival (even with the tissue).
3. Subgingival.

Q3. Which types of margins are best from periodontal point of view?

Answer

Supragingival margins have the least impact on the periodontium. The use of equigingival margins was thought to retain more plaque thereby interfering with gingival health; today these concerns are not valid. The greatest biologic risk occurs when margins are placed subgingivally. Hence, from periodontal point of view, both supragingival and equigingival margins are well tolerated.

Q4. Where are the restorative margins should be placed?

Answer

Restorative margins should be preferably placed supragingivally. However, in certain situations, where subgingival margins are unavoidable like carious tooth, tooth fracture or esthetic concern, it should be placed not more than 0.5 mm into the sulcus so that, these margins could be accessible for finishing procedures. If the margins are placed too far below the gingival tissue crest, it violates the gingival attachment apparatus.

Q5. What are the rules for margin placement?

Answer

Rule 1

If the probing depth is 1.5 mm or less, the restoration margin has to be placed below gingival tissue crest.

Rule 2

If the probing depth is more than 1.5 mm, then the margin of the restoration is placed at one-half of the probing depth below the gingival crest.

Rule 3

If the sulcus probing depth is more than 2 mm, then the tooth has to be evaluated for gingivectomy procedure to reduce the sulcus depth to 1.5 mm. Once this is achieved, margin placement is done in accordance to rule 1.

Q6. Why restorative margins should not invade into biologic width?

Answer

Invasion into this biologic width should be avoided in order to prevent attachment loss and persistent gingival inflammation.

Q7. What are the methods to correct biological width violation?

Answer

Biological width violation can be corrected either surgically (removing bone away from proximity to the restorative margin) or orthodontically (by moving the tooth and thus moving the margin away from the bone).

The orthodontic procedure can be accomplished in two ways:
1. *By slow orthodontic extrusive force:* The tooth is extruded by slowly bringing the bone and gingival tissue with it.
2. *By rapid orthodontic extrusive force:* Where the tooth extrusion to the desired amount is carried out over several weeks.

Q8. What are the requirements for ideal tooth contour?
Answer

An ideal contour must provide:
1. Access for hygiene.
2. Fullness to create the desired gingival form.
3. Esthetically pleasing tooth contour.
4. Protection of the marginal gingiva from mechanical injury during mastication—explained in gingival protection theory.

Hence, the crown contour should therefore help in easy plaque removal, not its retention. Overcontouring leads to more plaque accumulation with subsequent gingival inflammation under contouring of crowns, and therefore considered ideal.

Q9. Why are proper interproximal contour and embrasure necessary?
Answer

It is believed that the ideal interproximal embrasure should house the gingival papilla without impinging on it. Proper proximal contact is essential to prevent food impaction. The contact point should be placed occlusally and facially to facilitate access for interproximal plaque control. The ideal contact should be 2–3 mm coronal to the attachment, which coincides with the depth of the average interproximal sulcus.

Q10. What are the different types of pontic design?
Answer

Traditionally, four types of pontic designs have been proposed—sanitary, ridge lap, modified ridge lap and ovate pontic designs, which are detailed as follows:
1. *Sanitary pontic:* Where the tissue surface of the pontic is 3 mm from the underlying ridge.
2. *Ridge lap pontic:* Where the tissue surface of the pontic straddles the ridge much like a saddle. The entire surface is convex and is very difficult to clean.
3. *Modified ridge lap pontic:* The tissue surface on the facial surface is concave; however, the lingual saddle has been removed to allow access for oral hygiene.
4. *Ovate pontic:* This is the ideal pontic design. It is created by forming a receptor site in the edentulous ridge with either a diamond bur or electrosurgery.

Q11. What is the sequence of treatment in preparing periodontium for restorative dentistry?
Answer

It can be divided into two phases:
1. Control of active periodontal inflammation with non-surgical and surgical treatment:
    a. Extraction of hopeless teeth.
    b. Scaling, root planing and oral hygiene instructions.
    c. Re-evaluation, anti-infective therapy.
    d. Periodontal surgery.
    e. Adjunctive orthodontic therapy.
2. Preprosthetic surgery:
    a. Treatment of mucogingival deformities.
    b. Ridge reconstruction and preservation.
    c. Crown lengthening procedure.

Q12. What is biologic width?
Answer

The soft tissue attachment to the tooth between the base of the gingival sulcus and the crest of the alveolar bone is called biologic width.

CHAPTER 55

Drugs Used in Periodontal Therapy

Q1. Classify various drugs used in the periodontal therapy.

Answer

Various drugs used in periodontal therapy can be divided into:
1. Antiplaque and anticalculus agents.
2. Antibiotics in the management of periodontal disease.
3. Anti-inflammatory drugs.

Q2. Classify the various drugs used depending on antimicrobial efficacy and substantivity.

Answer

Depending on antimicrobial efficacy and substantivity drugs can be classified as:
1. *First-generation agents:* They reduce plaque score by 20%–50%, efficacy is limited because of poor substantivity.
   For example, antibiotics, quaternary ammonium compounds and sanguinarine. It should be used 4–6 times daily.
2. *Second-generation agents:* They are retained longer in the tissues and their slow-release property provides overall reduction in plaque score by 70%–90% (should be used twice daily).
   For example, chlorhexidine, triclosan with either copolymer or zinc citrate.
3. *Third-generation agents:* It should be effective against specific periodontopathic organisms. The most promising agent seems to be delmopinol, which is a surface-active agent. Though it is a weak antimicrobial agent, it can exert its effect by binding to salivary proteins and thereby alters the cohesive and adhesive properties of the films formed.

Q3. What are chemotherapeutic agents?

Answer

Chemotherapeutic agents refer to the ability of an active chemical substance to provide a therapeutic clinical benefit.

Q4. What are antimicrobials?

Answer

Antimicrobial agents are chemotherapeutic agents that reduce the amount of bacteria present either by specifically targeting certain organisms or by non-specifically reducing all bacteria.

Q5. What are antibiotics?

Answer

Antibiotics are a form of antimicrobial agents produced by or obtained from microorganisms that have the capacity to kill other microorganisms or inhibit their growth.

Q6. What are the advantages of systemic medication?

Answer

1. It ensures drug penetration till the base of the pocket.
2. Affects tissue invasive organisms.
3. Takes less time and is inexpensive.
4. Treats multiple sites simultaneously.
5. In acute conditions like necrotizing ulcerative gingivitis (NUG), etc. it is used to decrease active inflammation.
6. As a premedication for patients with medical problems requiring prophylactic antibiotic coverage.

Q7. What are the advantages of local drug administration?

Answer

1. Greater concentrations are achieved with reduced drug doses.
2. Systemic side effects are reduced.
3. Slow-releasing devices have the advantage of releasing antibiotics gradually.
4. Their effect can be directed to specific target area.

Q8. What are the requirements for an ideal antibiotic in periodontics according to Gibson?

Answer

According to Gibson, an ideal antibiotic for use in prevention and treatment of periodontal diseases should be:
- Specific to periodontal pathogens
- Allogenic
- Non-toxic, substantive
- Not in general use for treatment of other diseases
- Inexpensive.

Q9. Why is tetracycline used in treatment of periodontal diseases?

Answer

Tetracycline antibiotics are bacteriostatic and are generally more effective against gram-positive bacteria than gram-negative bacteria. Tetracyclines are very effective in treating periodontal diseases mainly because of their concentration in gingival crevicular fluid (GCF), which is 2–10 times more than that in serum. In addition, many studies have proved that tetracyclines even at low concentrations are very effective against many periodontal pathogens.

Q10. What are the other properties of tetracyclines, which are of value in the management of periodontal diseases?

Answer

1. *Tetracyclines and collagenase inhibition (host-derived collagenase):* These enzymes are derived from a variety of sources including fibroblasts, epithelial cells, macrophages and neutrophils. Collagenases derived from neutrophils are more susceptible to tetracycline induced inhibition.
2. *Tetracyclines and bone resorption:* The antiproteolytic properties together with anticollagenase activity have resulted in the use of these drugs to stop/inhibit bone resorption. Tetracyclines also inhibit bone resorption induced by parathyroid hormone, prostaglandin E series and bacterial endotoxins.
3. *Anti-inflammatory actions of tetracyclines:* Potential anti-inflammatory properties include the ability of tetracyclines to suppress polymorphonuclear leukocyte activity, in particular, the scavenging action of reactive oxygen metabolites. Alternatively, the drugs may block eicosanoid synthesis (PGE_2) by inhibiting phospholipase A_2 activity.
4. *Tetracycline and fibroblast attachment:*
   a. Pretreatment of dentin with tetracyclines enhances fibroblast attachment and colonization. Tetracycline can both condition the root surface and influence the attachment properties of fibroblasts.
   b. Tetracyclines can bind to demineralize and release from dentin. The substantivity of tetracycline is proportional to the concentration of the drug rather than to the time of application.
   c. The drug also enhances fibronectin binding.

Q11. What are the adverse effects of tetracyclines?

Answer

1. *Gastrointestinal disturbances:*
   - Diarrhea
   - Nausea and vomiting
   - Severe colitis (rare).
2. *Overgrowth of resistant organisms:*
   - Stomatitis
   - Vaginitis
   - Staphylococcal enterocolitis.
3. *Photosensitivity:*
   - Skin rashes
   - Hypersensitivity reactions.

Q12. What are the contraindications for the use of tetracyclines?

Answer

1. *Pregnancy*—staining of deciduous teeth, impaired bone growth.
2. *Breastfeeding*—staining of developing teeth and gastrointestinal disturbance in children.
3. *Renal impairment*—aggravates uremia.
4. *Hepatic disease.*
5. *Systemic lupus erythematosus*—exacerbation of lesions.

Q13. What is the dosage of tetracycline?

Answer

Tetracycline: Requires administration of 250 mg four times a day. It is inexpensive, but compliance may be reduced by taking four capsules a day.

Q14. What is the dosage of minocycline?

Answer

Minocycline: Exhibits broad spectrum of antibacterial activity especially in patients with adult periodontitis.

Dosage: 200 mg twice a day for 1 week, side effects include reversible vertigo.

Q15. What is the dosage of doxycycline?

Answer

Doxycycline: Same spectrum of activity as minocycline. Absorption from gastrointestinal tract is not altered by calcium, metal ions or antacids.

Dosage: 100 mg twice on the 1st day followed by 100 mg once a day or 50 mg twice a day for 4 days.

Q16. What is the dosage of metronidazole?

Answer

Dosage: 200 mg four times a day for 1 week or 400 mg three times a day for 1 week.

Q17. What are the side effects of metronidazole?

Answer

1. It has Antabuse effect when alcohol is ingested.
2. The symptoms include severe cramps, nausea and vomiting.
3. It inhibits warfarin metabolism.
4. Patients on anticoagulant therapy should avoid this drug because it prolongs prothrombin time.

Q18. What is the mechanism of action of NSAID?

Answer

After the activation of inflammatory cells in the periodontium by bacteria, phospholipids in the plasma membranes of cells are activated by the enzyme phospholipase A_2 and this leads to release of free arachidonic acid in the area. Arachidonic acid can then be metabolized into prostaglandins, thromboxanes and prostacyclins by cyclooxygenase or into leukotrienes, HETE and SRS-A by lipoxygenase enzyme. NSAIDs work by inhibiting both cyclooxygenase 1 and cyclooxygenase 2, or by selectively inhibiting cyclooxygenase 2 pathway. Therefore, providing anti-inflammatory, analgesic and antipyretic effect.

Q19. What are the indications for local drug delivery system?

Answer

1. As an adjunct in the treatment of few localized non-responding sites in an otherwise controlled patient.
2. In ailing and failing implant cases.
3. In medically compromised patients where surgical procedures are not recommended.
4. Periodontal abscess.
5. Periodontal maintenance therapy.
6. Patient with gastrointestinal intolerance to systemic drug medication.

Q20. What are the contraindications for local drug delivery system?

Answer

1. Patients with history of allergy to a particular antimicrobial agent.
2. In pregnancy and lactating periods.
3. Children under the age of 12 years.
4. Patients with complete renal failure.
5. Patients susceptible to infective endocarditis.

Q21. What are the vehicles for local delivery of chemotherapeutic agents?

Answer

Dentifrices, mouthrinses, chewing gum and slow-release devices.

Q22. What are slow-release devices/controlled-release delivery systems?

Answer

The systems are designed to release chemotherapeutic agents into the periodontal pocket over an extended period of time; hence they can achieve high levels of concentration at sites where they are precisely needed.

Q23. Classify controlled-release local delivery systems.

Answer

1. Reservoirs without a rate-controlling system, e.g. hollow fibers, gels and dialysis tubing (effective only for 24 hour).
2. Reservoirs with a rate-controlling system, e.g. polymeric matrices, polymer membranes, monolithic matrices and coated particles (effective for more than 24 hour).

Q24. What is the ethylene-vinyl acetate (EVA) system?

Answer

EVA system is based on polymer technology with tetracycline dispersed within a solid (monolithic) polymer of EVA. A formulation of 25% tetracycline in EVA (Actisite) has been developed as 0.5 mm non-biodegradable fiber and has been approved by the Food and Drug Administration (FDA).

Q25. What are the methods of delivery of chemotherapeutic agents?

Answer

1. Keyes technique.
2. Root biomodification.
3. Irrigation devices.
    a. Home irrigation devices:
        - Supragingival home irrigation devices
        - Subgingival home irrigation devices
        - Marginal home irrigation devices.
    b. Professional subgingival irrigation.

Q26. Describe the Keyes technique.

Answer

Involves application, by toothbrushing, of slurry of sodium bicarbonate and hydrogen peroxide for the control of plaque microorganisms. Various studies have proved that minimal clinical benefit can be expected from this technique simply because toothbrushing offers an ineffective means of delivering medicaments into the periodontal pocket.

Q27. Name some locally delivered antimicrobials for periodontal therapy.

Answer

Trade name	Antimicrobial agent
Actisite	Tetracycline
Atridox	Doxycycline
Arestin	Minocycline
Dentomycin	Minocycline
Elyzol	Metronidazole
PerioChip	Chlorhexidine
Atrigel	5% sanguinarine

Index

Page numbers followed by *f* refer to figure and *t* refer to table.

A

Acellular
  afibrillar cementum, 43
  cementum, 43
Acquired immunodeficiency syndrome, 100
Acteroides forsythus, 154
Actinomycetemcomitans, 99
Acute
  bleeding, 73
  gingival infections, 82
  herpetic gingivostomatitis, 84
  infection, role in, 57
  necrotizing ulcerative gingivitis, 76, 82
Addison's disease, 74
Addy's classification, 127
Aggregatibacter actinomycetemcomitans, 65, 111
Aggressive periodontitis, 98
AHG
  signs of, 84
  symptoms of, 84
AIDS
  and periodontium, 102
  including advanced diagnostic aids, 109
Albright's disease, 74
Alloplast, 142
Alloplastic, management of, 158
Alveolar
  bone, 43, 45, 86
  gingival fibers, 42
Ambulatory patients, treatment for, 84
Amelogenin, 38
American Academy of Periodontology, 72
Anemia, 74
Angiogranuloma, 79
Angular defects, 95
Antibodies, 66
Anti-inflammatory
  actions of tetracyclines, 169
  cytokines, 65
Antimicrobial agents, classification of, 127
ANUG, treatment for, 83
Arch fulcrum, 120
Ascorbic acid, 61
Attached gingiva
  amount of, 10
  width of, 39
Azurophilic granules, contents of, 57

B

Bacteria in ANUG, role of, 83
Bacterial
  complexes, types of, 52
  zone, 83
Bacteroides
  forsythus, 101
  intermedius, 83
BANA test, 111
Basal lamina, 40
Benzoyl-DL-arginine-naphthylamide, 64
Biochemical diagnosis, 111
Biofilm, 51
  features of, 51
Bleeding on probing, 10
Blood supply of gingiva, 41
Bone
  blend, 142
  defects, 95
  destruction
    in periodontal disease, 94
    patterns of, 94
    patterns, types of, 95
  grafts, 137
    sources of, 143
  implant interfaces, 158
  loss, 94
    horizontal, 95
  regeneration, 140
  swaging, 142
    disadvantages of, 143
Brushite, 53
Burtonian line, 74

C

Calcium, 53
  phosphate ceramics, types of, 143
Calculocementum, 53
Calculus, 53
  composition of, 53
  formation of, 53
  significance of, 54
  types of, 53
Capnocytophaga, 52, 80
Carbonate, 53
Caustic drugs, 132
CEJ, detection of, 12*f*
Cell, 40
  protein, 65
Cellular cementum, 43
Cementoenamel junction, 75
Cementum, 43, 45, 86
  composition of, 43
  functions of, 43
Cervical enamel projections, 149
Charter's method, 126
Chédiak-Higashi syndrome, 62
Chemosurgery, disadvantages of, 134
Chemotherapeutic agents, 168
  delivery of, 170
Chisel scaler, 24, 116
  design, 24
  uses, 24
Chronic
  bleeding, 73
  desquamative gingivitis, 88
  gingivitis, 74
  granulomatous disease, 62

obstructive pulmonary disease, 67
  periodontitis, 19, 96
Citric acid, actions of, 141
Civatte bodies, 89
Clock positions for right-handed clinician, 30*f*
Co-aggregation, 51
Collagen splicing, 141
Colloidal proteins, 54
Color-coded probes, 114
Conventional periodontal probes, types of, 109
Correct finger placement, 32*t*
Crevicular incision, 136
Cross-arch fulcrum, 120
Crystal forms, 53
Cumine scaler, 24
  use, 24
Curette
  characteristics of, 25
  parts of, 26*f*
  types of, 115
  uses of, 114
Curved scaler, design of, 23*f*
Cyclic neutropenia, 61
Cyclosporin, 78
Cytokines, 65, 66

D

Defense mechanism
  of gingiva, 70
  types of, 70
Dental
  floss
    choice of, 127
    types of, 127
  implants: periodontal considerations, 158
  light, 30
  mirror, uses of, 119
  plaque, 51
    formation of, 52
    types of, 51
  splinting, 156
Dentogingival
  fibers, 42
  unit, 40
Dentoperiodontal unit, 39
Dentoperiosteal fibers, 42
Desmosome, composition of, 41
Desquamative gingivitis, 88
Diabetes, 107
  mellitus, treatment in, 63
Diagnostic instruments, 21
Diamond probe, 64
Direct visibility, 30*f*
Disease process, changes in consistency, 74
DNA probes, 111
  in identification of periodontal pathogens, 111
Double papilla flap, 146
  advantages of, 146
Down syndrome, 104

Doxycycline, dosage of, 169
Drugs used in periodontal therapy, 168

E

Enamel epithelium, 38
Enameloids, 38
Endoperiolesions, 154
Endotoxin, 65
Enlargement in pregnancy, types of, 79
Envelope technique, 147
Epithelial cells, 41
Epstein-Barr virus, 84
Essential oil rinse, 128
Ethylene vinyl acetate system, 116
Exaggerated scalloping, 7f
Extraoral fulcrum, 121

F

Familial neutropenia, 62
Fanconi's anemia, effect of, 63
Fibers, 40
Finger
    on finger, 33f
        fulcrum, 121
    rest, 32
Flap
    after surgery, placement of, 135
    procedure and gingivectomy, comparison between, 137
Fluoride, 53
Fones technique, disadvantage of, 126
Free nerve endings, 42
Free soft tissue autograft
    advantages of, 144
    disadvantages of, 144
Freeze-dried bone allograft, 143, 152
    demineralized, 143
Fremitus, clinical demonstration of, 14
Frenal attachments, types of, 148
Frenectomy, 148
Frenotomy, 148
Frenum, 148
Furcation
    defects, 149, 150
    entrance, detection of, 14f
    examination, 13, 14f
    fornix, 153
    involvement, 149
    management, 149
    to Goldman, classify, 150
Fusobacterium nucleatum, 52

G

Gas chromatography, 64
Gas-liquid chromatography, 111
Gastrointestinal
    disturbances, 169
    tract, diseases of, 64
Gender, 107
General health and gingival fluid, 71
Generalized periodontitis, 96
Genetic factors, 99
Gingipains, 65
Gingiva, 37, 45
    changes in, 86
    color of, 37
    contour of, 74
    in disease, position of, 9f
    in gingiva exhibiting rolled margins with blunt papillae, examination of, 7t
    normal size of, 8f
Gingival
    autograft, 146
    bleeding, 73
        systemic causes of, 73
    bone count index, 49
    crevicular fluid, 56, 70, 169
    curettage, 131
    disease, 48
    enlargement, 77
        combined, 79
    epithelium, 41
    fibers, functions of, 41
    inflammation, 72
        signs of, 73
    lesions, 86
    recession, 145
        position of, 9f
        prognosis of, 145
    status, 2
        periodontal charting, 2
    tumors, 77
Gingivectomy, 133
    indications of, 133
    prerequisites of, 133
    used for, 134
Gingivitis, 46, 72
    classify, 73
    clinical features of, 73
    treatment of, 18
Gingivoplasty, 133
Glickman's
    bone factor, 95
    concept, 59
    furcation classification, 14
Goals of suturing, 130
Gracey
    and universal curettes, distinction between, 115
    curettes, 122
    instrument series, 115
Gradualizing marginal bone, 139
Grasps, types of, 119
GTR technique, 147
Guided tissue regeneration, 68, 141

H

Handle, types of, 21
Hard tissue examination, 10
Hemidesmosomes, pairs of, 41
Herpes virus type 1, 84
Hertwig's epithelial root sheath, 37
Heterograft, 142
HIV infection, 102
HIV/acquired immunodeficiency syndrome, 108
Hoe scalers, 24, 116
    design of, 24
    types, 24
    use, 24
Hopewell-Smith or intermediate cementum, layer of, 38
Host modulation in periodontal therapy, 69
Host response: basic concepts, 56
Host-derived collagenase, 169
Human immunodeficiency virus infections, 102
Hyaline layer of Hopewell-Smith, 44
Hydroxyapatite, 53

I

Idiopathic gingival fibromatosis, 79
Iliac autografts, disadvantages of, 143
Immune responses, 65, 66
Implants, types of, 158
Indications of electrosurgery, 134
Indirect visibility, 30f
Inflammatory gingival enlargement, 9f, 78
Infrabony pockets, 13, 92
Infrequent dental visits, 108
Inorganic component of calculus, 53
Instrument
    activation, 32
    adaptation in
        embrasure area, 34f
        posterior embrasure area, 34f
    adaptation on lower anteriors, 34f
    angulation, 33f
    grasps, 31
    parts of, 21f
    sharpness
        advantages of, 30
        condition of, 30
    stabilization, 31
    strokes, types of, 34f
Intercuspal position, 162
Interdental
    brushes, 127
    gingiva, 37
Internal bevel incision, 136
Interproximal bone, 139
    indicated, 139
Inter-radicular and interdental arteries, 42
Intraoral
    and extraoral finger rests, 32
    autograft, 142
    finger rests, 120
    fulcrum, 120
Islet scaler, 25
    use, 25

J

Jacquette scaler, design of, 23f
Jaundice, 74
Junctional epithelium, length of, 40
Juvenile periodontitis, 97

K

Keratinosomes, 41
Knuckle-rest technique or palm up technique, 121

L

Lamina propria, 40
Langer and Langer technique, 147
Langer's technique, 147
Laterally displaced flap, advantages of, 145
Lazy Leukocyte syndrome, 62
Lesions, distribution of, 98
Leukemia, 62, 74
    manifestations of, 62
Leukemic patients, treatment plan for, 62
Lichen planus, 89
Lipooligosaccharide, 65
Lipopolysaccharides, 68
Local causes, 42

Index

Localized
    and generalized periodontitis, differentiate between, 96
    periodontitis, 96

M

Magnesium, 53
    whitlockite, 53
Mandibular teeth, light position for, 31*f*
Marginal gingiva in health, position of, 9*f*
Marquis color-coded probe, 109, 114
Maxillary teeth, light position for, 31*f*
McCall's festoons, 76
Meissener's corpuscles, 42
Metronidazole
    dosage of, 170
    side effects of, 170
Miller's classification, 145
Mini langer curettes, 115
Minocycline, dosage of, 169
Mirror surfaces, types of, 118
Missing first molar, 59
Mobility
    causes of, 103
    clinical demonstration of, 14*f*
Morse scaler, 23
    design, 23
    uses, 23
Mouth mirror, 21
    design, 21
    sizes, 21
    surfaces, types of, 118
    uses, 21
Mouthwash, properties of, 127
Mucogingival
    junction, 37
    surgery, 144

N

Necrotizing ulcerative
    gingivitis, 82, 100, 168
    periodontitis, 100
Neutral
    back position, 28*f*
    forearm position, 28*f*
    hand position, 29*f*
    neck position, 27*f*
    seated position for clinician, 27*f*
    shoulder position, 28*f*
    upper arm position, 28*f*
Neutropenia, 104
    of childhood, 62
    types of, 61
Neutrophil-rich zone, 83
Nifedipine, 78
Nikolsky's sign, 88
Non-ambulatory patients, treatment for, 83
Non-color-coded probes, 114
Non-Hodgkin's lymphoma, 102
Non-keratinized epithelium, 40
Non-oxidative mechanism, 57
Non-specific plaque hypothesis, 52
Normal color of gingiva, 73
NUG
    names of, 82
    signs of, 82
    symptoms of, 82

O

Octacalcium phosphate, 53
Odland bodies, 41
Ole of macrophages in development, 56
Opposite arch, 33*f*
Opsonization, 56
Oral
    epithelium, 39
    implantology, 158
    lesions associated with HIV infection, 102
    malodor, 64
    mucosa, 45
    symptoms, 82
Orogranulocytes, 70
Orthodontic
    adjunct to periodontal therapy, role of, 164
    treatment, 164
Orthokeratinization, 40
Osseointegration, 158
Osseous
    coagulum, 142
        disadvantages of, 142
    resective surgery, 138
    reshaping, definitive, 138
    surgery, 138
        definition of, 138
        types of, 138
Osteoinduction, 142
Ovate pontic, 167
Oxygen-dependent killing mechanism, 57

P

P. gingivalis, 111
Paget's disease, 42
Palm and thumb grasp, 31*f*, 119
Palm
    down, 32*f*
    up, 32*f*
Papilla
    management of, 135
    preservation flap, 136
Papillon-Lefevre syndrome, 57
Parakeratinization, 40
Pathologic tooth migration, 59
Pen grasp, 31*f*
    modified, 119, 31*f*
Peri-implant
    diseases, types of, 158
    mucositis, 158
Peri-implantitis, 159
Periodontains, 66
Periodontal
    diseases, 57, 61, 65, 107
        causes for recurrence of, 160
        classification systems of, 46
        diagnosis of, 103
        in breastfeeding, 63
        in children and young adolescents, 86
        indicators of, 108
        management of, 162
        progression of, 59
    examination, 11
    file, 24
        design, 24
        uses, 25
    flap, 135
    instrumentation, 21, 114
        classification of, 21
        parts of, 21
        principles of, 26
    lesions, 86
    ligament, 42, 86
        functions of, 43
    manifestations, 62
    medicine, 67
    microbiology, 51
    pocket, 90
        formation, 91
        probing, 11
    probes, 22, 22*f*, 109
        design, 22
        generations of, 22
        shank, 22
        types of, 22, 114
        uses of, 22
    restorative inter-relationship, 166
    screening and recording, 110
    splint, 156
    structures in aging humans, 45
    surgeries, 68
    surgery, 135
        principles of, 129
    therapy, 160, 168
        treatment in, 164
    tissues, 58
        biology of, 39
    treatment, 160, 164
        plan, 17, 18*f*
Periodontia, 37
Periodontics, 37
Periodontitis, 46
Periodontium, 39
Periodontium
    anatomy of structures of, 37
    components of, 37
    development of structures of, 37
    normal surface characteristics of, 6*f*
Peutz-Jeghers disease, 74
Phenytoin, 78
Phosphorus, 53
Physiologic halitosis, causes of, 64
Piggy-backed fulcrum, 120
Pitting on pressure with disease, 8*f*
Plak-lite system, 128
Plaque
    composition of, 51
    control, 124
        measures, 124
    hypothesis, 52
    pathogenic, 52
Plasma cell gingivitis, 80
Platelet-derived growth factor, 143
Platelet-rich fibrin, 143
Pocket
    epithelium, 140
    therapy, techniques for, 136
    treatment of, 92
    types of, 12
Polyacrylamide gel electrophoresis, 111
Polymorphonuclear
    leukocytes, 65, 99
    neutrophil, 61
Pontic design, types of, 167
Porphyromonas gingivalis, 52, 65, 154
Position of gingiva, 75
Pouch and tunnel technique, 147
Powered toothbrushes, 126
Pregnancy
    tumor, 79
    marginal enlargement in, 79
Prevotella intermedia, 52, 83, 111, 165
Pristine gingiva, 72
Probe
    different types of, 22*f*
    in perpendicular position, 12*f*
Procedure with gingivectomy, 137
Progenitor cells, 41
Prognosis and risk, differences between, 105

Proinflammatory cytokines, 65
Prostaglandins, 66
Protrusion, 162
Pubertal gingival enlargement, 80
Pulp and periodontium, communication between, 154
Pulpoperiodontal problems, 154

Q

Quéntin furcation curettes, 116

R

Radiographic AIDS, advanced, 110
Rapid orthodontic extrusive force, 167
Rate of plaque formation, 51
Rationale for periodontal treatment, 113
Recession
    classification of, 75
    types of, 75
Recurrent and refractory periodontitis, distinction between, 101
Refractory periodontitis, 100
Regeneration, 113
Remodeling of periodontium, 58
Removal of pocket wall, 93
Resorptive cells, 41
Retraction, 30
Ridge lap pontic, 167
    modified, 167
Right submandibular lymph node, palpation of, 5f
Root
    biomodification, 141
    complex, parts of, 152
    coverage procedures, advantages of, 145
    planing instruments, 25
        advances in, 25
    resorption, 165
    separation, 152
    trunk, 152
Ruffini-like mechanoreceptors, 42
RUG delivery system, 170

S

Saliva, functions of, 71
Sample periodontal chart, 13, 13f
Sanitary pontic, 167
Scaler and curette, differences between, 26
Scaling
    and root planing instruments, 23
    instruments, 23
Scoring criteria for
    CI-S, 50
    DI-S, 49
Scrub technique, 126
Semilunar flap, disadvantages of, 146
Shank, types of, 21
Sharpey's fibers, 38
Sickle scaler, 23
    cross section of, 114
    design, 23, 23f
    functions, 23
Smoking
    and periodontal disease, 68
    on gingivitis, 68
    on immune system, 68
    on periodontitis, 68
    on periodontium, 68

Sodium, 53
Sorrin's classification of habits, 55
Splints
    classify, 156
    in periodontal therapy, 156
Stages
    in neutrophil chemotaxis, 56
    of gingivitis, 72
Staphylococcus intermedius, 101
Stillman's
    cleft, 8f
    method, 125
    technique, 125
Stippling
    cause of, 75
    in disease, absence of, 9f
    with healthy gingiva, normal, 9f
Straight scaler, design of, 23f
Stratum
    basale, 39
    corneum, 39
    germinativum, 39
    granulosum, 39
    spinosum, 39
Streptococcus sanguinis, 52
Stroke
    by direction, types of, 33
    characteristics of, 34t
    directions, types of, 122
    types of, 121
Subclinical gingivitis, 72
Subepithelial connective tissue graft, 147
Subgingival
    curettage, 131
    plaque, 51
    scalers, 23, 24, 25
Subpopulation of fibroblasts, 78
Sulcus bleeding index, 49
Supine patient position, 29f
Supportive periodontal treatment, 160
Suprabony pockets, 12, 92
Supracrestal gingival fibers, 60
Supragingival
    and subgingival calculus, differences between, 54
    plaque, 51
    scalers, 23
Surface scaler, 24
    use, 24
Surgery, principles of, 129
Suturing materials, 130
Syndrome
    Chédiak-Higashi, 62
    Down, 104
    Lazy Leukocyte, 62
    Papillon-Lefevre, 57
Synthetic cells, 41
Systemic
    causes, 42
    disease, manifestation of, 100
    medication, advantages of, 168

T

Tetracycline
    and bone resorption, 169
    and collagenase inhibition, 169
    and fibroblast attachment, 169
    dosage of, 169
    use of, 169

Texture of gingiva, 75
TFO, symptoms of, 58
Tissue
    management, 130
    response to periodontal therapy, 19
TMJ
    palpation of, 5f
    with fingers placed behind condyle, palpation of, 5f
Tobacco smoking, 107
Tooth
    contour, 167
    in furcation defects, 149
    migration, 59
Toothbrush
    design of, 124
    specifications of, 124
Traditional treatment procedure, 151
Transforming growth factor-beta, 141
Transillumination, 30
Transseptal fibers, 42
Trauma from occlusion, 58
Trial maintenance therapy, 160
True pockets, measurement of, 12
Tzanck cells, 89

U

Ultrasonic
    and sonic instruments, types of, 116
    scalers, types of, 123
    vibrations, frequency of, 116
Universal
    and gracey curettes, differences between, 26
    curettes, 115, 122
Urinary glucose, 63

V

Varicella zoster virus, 84
Vitamin
    B, deficiency of, 61
    D deficiency, 61
Volatile sulfur compounds, 64
Volume of GCF, 70

W

Waerhaug's measurements, 94
White blood cell disorders, 61
Widman flap, 136
Widow's peaks, 139
Working end of
    area-specific curette, 27f
    chisel, 24f
    file, 24f
    hoe, 24f
    scaler, 26f
    types of, 21
    universal curette, 27f

X

Xenograft, 142

Z

Zone of spirochetal infiltration, 83